The Language of Mental Health

Series Editors
Michelle O'Reilly
The Greenwood Institute
University of Leicester
Leicester, UK

Jessica Nina Lester
School of Education
Indiana University Bloomington
Bloomington, IN, USA

This series brings together rich theoretical and empirical discussion at the intersection of mental health and discourse/conversation analysis. Situated broadly within a social constructionist perspective, the books included within this series will offer theoretical and empirical examples highlighting the discursive practices that surround mental health and make 'real' mental health constructs. Drawing upon a variety of discourse and conversation analysis perspectives, as well as data sources, the books will allow scholars and practitioners alike to better understand the role of language in the making of mental health. Editorial board We are very grateful to our expert editorial board who continue to provide support for the book series. We are especially appreciative of the feedback that they have provided on earlier drafts of this book. Their supportive comments and ideas to improve the book have been very helpful in our development of the text. They continue to provide support as we continue to edit the book series 'the language of mental health'. We acknowledge them here in alphabetical order by surname.

More information about this series at
http://www.palgrave.com/gp/series/15193

Olga Smoliak • Tom Strong
Editors

Therapy as Discourse

Practice and Research

palgrave
macmillan

Editors
Olga Smoliak
University of Guelph
Guelph, ON, Canada

Tom Strong
University of Calgary
Calgary, AB, Canada

The Language of Mental Health
ISBN 978-3-030-06578-2 ISBN 978-3-319-93067-1 (eBook)
https://doi.org/10.1007/978-3-319-93067-1

Cover illustration: g-stockstudio\gettyimages

This Palgrave Macmillan imprint is published by the registered company Springer Nature Switzerland AG
The registered company address is: Gewerbestrasse 11, 6330 Cham, Switzerland

Contents

Notes on Contributors

Evrinomy Avdi, PhD, is an Associate Professor in Clinical Psychology at the School of Psychology of the Aristotle University of Thessaloniki, Greece. She is a clinical psychologist, psychodynamic psychotherapist, and drama therapist. Her research interests lie in applying discursive and narrative research to the study of the process of psychotherapy, as well as the experience of serious illness. She is particularly interested in exploring the links between deconstructive research and actual clinical practice.

Jessica ChenFeng, PhD, is a liberative educator and therapist who focuses on issues of gender, culture, spirituality, and power in her clinical work and research. As an Assistant Professor of Marriage and Family Therapy (MFT) in the Department of Educational Psychology and Counseling at California State University, Northridge, she enjoys supporting students toward whole-person development. She is a second-generation Taiwanese American woman residing in the San Gabriel Valley of Los Angeles, hoping for and working toward cross-generational/racial/disciplinary transformation.

Shari Couture, PhD, is a psychologist and family therapist working in private practice in Calgary, Alberta, Canada. She has been a clinical supervisor of family therapy students at the Family Therapy Centre in Calgary and currently is an instructor for the Master in Counselling Program at the University of Calgary. As a researcher, she discursively analyzes the process of therapy.

Robert Elliott, PhD, is a Professor of Counselling at the University of Strathclyde, Scotland. He received his PhD in Clinical Psychology from the

University of California, Los Angeles, where he also studied conversation analysis with Manny Schegloff. Before moving to Scotland in 2006, he was a Professor of Clinical Psychology at the University of Toledo (Ohio). He is a co-author of *Facilitating Emotional Change* (1993), *Learning Emotion-Focused Psychotherapy* (2004), and *Research Methods in Clinical Psychology* (2014) and in more than 150 journal articles and book chapters. In 2008, he received the Distinguished Research Career Award from the Society for Psychotherapy Research and the Carl Rogers Award from the Division of Humanistic Psychology of the American Psychological Association. Over the years, he has drawn on conversation analysis (CA) in his research on significant therapy events and in his practice as a psychotherapist. He credits CA as one of the influences on the development of emotion-focused therapy (EFT).

Joaquín Gaete, PhD, is an Associate Professor, Clinical Supervisor, and Director of a Clinical Centre (CEAP) at Universidad Adolfo Ibáñez in Viña del Mar, Chile. His research and writing focus on conversational practices fostering self-preferred change in counseling, family therapy, and clinical supervision.

Aimee Galick, PhD, earned her doctoral degree in MFT in 2013. She was an Assistant Professor for three years before moving into a research analyst position for the Government of Alberta. She conducts research to support decision and policy making in post-secondary education. She continues to teach as an adjunct for the University of Louisiana Monroe and City University of Seattle. Her research interests include gender, couples therapy, and medical family therapy.

Eugenie Georgaca, PhD, is an Associate Professor in Clinical Psychology at the School of Psychology of the Aristotle University of Thessaloniki, Greece. She teaches, researches, and publishes in the area of clinical psychology, psychotherapy, and mental health and especially qualitative methodology, community mental health, and critical perspectives on psychopathology. She is a co-author of *Deconstructing Psychopathology* (Sage, 1995) and author of papers on psychotic discourse, delusions, discursive approaches to analyzing psychotherapy, discourse analysis, and social constructionist notions of subjectivity.

Adam O. Horvath, PhD, is a Professor Emeritus at Simon Fraser University. His research interests include the role and function of the relationship between therapist and clients in a variety of therapeutic settings. On the theoretical level, he is exploring the interactive processes that enable clients to generate new meaning of their problematic experiences, including the ones that brought them to therapy.

Carmen Knudson-Martin, PhD, is a Professor and Director of the Marital, Couple, and Family Therapy Program at Lewis & Clark College, Portland, OR. She has published over 80 articles and book chapters on the influence of the larger sociocultural context in couple and family relationships and the political and ethical implications of therapist actions. She is a founder of Socio-Emotional Relationship Therapy, an approach that bridges societal discourse, power, and couple interaction and a co-author of *Socioculturally Attuned Family Therapy: Guidelines for Equitable Theory and Practice.*

Elsie Lobo is a PhD candidate in the Marital and Family Therapy Program at Loma Linda University. She works primarily with couples and families at the Loma Linda Behavioral Health Institute where she also directs a clinic mentoring students in couples therapy. Elsie's research interests include seeking to understand how couples and families are shaped by social contexts, including gender, culture, and socio-economic status, and developing practices that attend to these contexts.

Gale Miller, PhD, is an Emeritus Professor of Sociology, Department of Social and Cultural Sciences, Marquette University. He has longstanding research interests in the Sociology of Troubles and Social Problems, Social Theory, and Social Institutions. His research has focused on how troubles and problems are defined in human service institutions, such as work to welfare programs and solution-focused brief therapy. His current research deals with individuals and families coping with such enduring crises as having a family member imprisoned for sex offenses in the United States as well as solution-focused brief therapy.

Peter Muntigl, PhD, is an Adjunct Professor in the Faculty of Education at Simon Fraser University, Canada, and a Visiting Research Professor in the Linguistics Department at Ghent University, Belgium. He is currently exploring how affiliation, disaffiliation, and re-affiliation are accomplished multi-modally during psychotherapy and family therapy interactions. His research is supported by the Social Sciences and Humanities Research Council of Canada.

Sarah K. Samman, CCRP, PMC-MedFT, PhD, is an Assistant Professor of Couple and Family Therapy at the California School of Professional Psychology, Alliant International University, San Diego. She has presented at national and international conferences on issues of gender and power on couple and family relationships. Sarah has a strong interdisciplinary background in health psychology and medical family therapy and has a deep commitment to social justice. She is an AAMFT Approved Supervisor.

Olga Smoliak, PhD, C. Psych., is an Associate Professor in Couple and Family Therapy at the University of Guelph. She has taken a social constructionist approach to psychotherapy and has explored the links between discourse and therapy. Olga has studied linguistic and interactional methods used by therapy participants to give and receive advice, collaborate, accomplish specific therapeutic tasks, and negotiate responsibility for blameworthy conduct. She is currently examining how therapists request in-session practical actions from clients and how the authority to direct clients' actions is interactionally implemented and negotiated.

William B. Stiles, PhD, is a Professor Emeritus of Psychology, Miami University, Oxford, Ohio, USA, and Adjunct Professor of Psychology at Appalachian State University, Boone, North Carolina, USA. He also taught at the University of North Carolina at Chapel Hill, and he has held visiting positions at the Universities of Sheffield and Leeds in the United Kingdom, at Massey University in New Zealand, at the University of Joensuu in Finland, and at Maia University Institute in Portugal. He received his PhD from UCLA in 1972. He has been President of Division 29 of the American Psychological Association (Society for the Advancement of Psychotherapy) and of the Society for Psychotherapy Research. He has served as an editor of *Psychotherapy Research* and *Person-Centered and Experiential Psychotherapies*. He has published more than 300 journal articles and book chapters, most dealing with psychotherapy, verbal interaction, and research methods.

Tom Strong, PhD, is a Professor, couple and family therapist, and counselor-educator at the University of Calgary who researches and writes on the collaborative, critically informed and practical potentials of discursive approaches to psychotherapy. His most recent book is *Medicalizing Counselling: Issues and Tensions* (Palgrave Macmillan). For more details on Tom, please consult http://www.ucalgary.ca/strongt or his ResearchGate page https://www.researchgate.net/profile/Tom_Strong.

Eleftheria Tseliou, PhD, is an Associate Professor of Research Methodology and Qualitative Methods at the University of Thessaly, Greece, and a systemic family psychotherapist. She teaches research methodology, qualitative methods, and family psychology. Her research interests include the development of discursive research methodologies and the study of psychotherapeutic and educational processes by discourse analysis methodology. She is an author of articles and book chapters on methodological aspects of discursive research methodologies and on family psychotherapy process studies. She is a co-editor (with Maria

Borcsa) of a special section on discursive methodologies for couple and family therapy research (*Journal of Marital and Family Therapy*).

Jarl Wahlström, PhD, is a Professor Emeritus in Clinical Psychology and Psychotherapy and former Director of the Psychotherapy Training and Research Centre at the Department of Psychology, University of Jyväskylä, Finland. He has served as the head of the national integrative postgraduate specialization program in psychotherapy for psychologists. He has an advanced training in family and systems therapy and an extensive experience as a clinical psychologist, family therapist, trainer, consultant, and university teacher. His main research interest is in psychotherapy discourse, a topic on which he has published in several international journals and books. He is the supervisor of several doctoral dissertations.

Kirstee Williams, PhD, is a Director and Assistant Professor for the Lee University Marriage and Family Therapy Program, the first COAMFTE-accredited program in the state of Tennessee. Her scholarship focuses on a social justice approach for infidelity treatment. Kirstee earned her doctorate in Marital and Family Therapy from Loma Linda University and is an active member in the American Family Therapy Academy.

1

Introduction to Discursive Research and Discursive Therapies

Tom Strong and Olga Smoliak

For more than a century, people have been referring to psychotherapy as the talking cure, with still vague understandings as to what it is about talking that is curative or therapeutic. What does talking have to do with how one understands and experiences reality? Why do therapists portray clients' concerns and solutions to them so differently? Such questions have prompted lots of theorizing by psychotherapists from often strikingly different orientations to practice. For those who turn to research for definitive answers, the results can often be similarly dissatisfying. The stance taken by discursive therapists and discursive researchers of therapy can perplex readers, especially if they overlook

T. Strong (✉)
Educational Studies in Counselling Psychology, Werklund School of Education, University of Calgary, Calgary, AB, Canada
e-mail: strongt@ucalgary.ca

O. Smoliak
Department of Family Relations and Applied Nutrition, University of Guelph, Guelph, ON, Canada
e-mail: osmoliak@uoguelph.ca

O. Smoliak, T. Strong (eds.), *Therapy as Discourse*, The Language of Mental Health,
https://doi.org/10.1007/978-3-319-93067-1_1

how language is used when representing and intervening in therapeutic realities.

Some of the perplexity might relate to therapeutic models' root metaphors (Pepper, 1942; Turnbull, 2003) for the foci and processes of therapeutic discourse in the first place. Are the concerns clients present, for example, about faulty information processing, ids needing taming, aversive childhood experiences, or dysfunctional patterns of relationships? What about therapeutic discourse or the talking between clients and therapists itself: are therapists doing forms of conversational surgery, can they administer conversational interventions in dosages, can good therapists engineer transformational experiences? These can seem silly questions to therapists and researchers who have taken up a discursive turn. For them, and for the authors of this volume, discourse is how humans negotiate and navigate socially constructed experiences, processes, concerns, and aspirations with each other. As for how all of this pertains to discursive researchers and therapists, their metaphors of interest relate to discourse as linguistically constructed meaning, and discourse as language use in human interactions.

If you are feeling uncomfortable reading about this language of metaphors as accounting for what is real, welcome to the club, but get used to it. Experiences and things do not name themselves; humans do and hold each other to account regarding the "right" or best ways to use language in describing those things and objects. To discursively informed practitioners and researchers, language use involves more than passive exchanges of information computed for accuracy and algorithmic decision-making (Ortega & Vidal, 2011). Important things are at stake over how language gets used, as debates over psychiatric diagnoses (e.g., Frances, 2013) underscore at a big picture level, but also in how therapists and clients wordsmith their ways forward in therapeutic conversation. Some see a more deferential thing occurring between client and therapist, where authoritative roles and expertise are to govern what gets talked about and how that talking is to occur (Rose, 1990). Beyond the consulting room, therapeutic discourse has found its way into people's everyday conversations and understandings—enough to have become a default discourse of self-understanding for many (Illouz, 2008).

Discourse, in the sense that most authors here will use the term, refers to conversational processes and meanings, without a sense that there is a "right" or more-real-than-others way to understand and humanly interact. Discourse, down to words, gestures, tones of voice (etc.), and their conversational use, is the focus of the work of psychotherapy. For discursive therapists, conversational work is needed to respond to the ways of understanding and communicating that clients bring in related to their concerns and aspirations, while negotiating changes to client problem or aspirational discourse. That work for discursive researchers is analyzable for what gets used in and is seen to result from therapeutic discourse.

Discursive approaches to therapy came into vogue in the 1980s. They drew on the linguistic insights of philosophers of science, like Wittgenstein (1953), Gadamer (1988), and Foucault (1973), but also the socio-political concerns of feminist (e.g., Weisstein, 1971) and postcolonial critics (e.g., Fanon, 1967). Inherent to the discursive approaches to therapy (primarily narrative, solution-focused, and collaborative therapy) is a view that meaning is socially constructed and that therapy itself is as a meaning-making/changing endeavor (McNamee & Gergen, 1992). Differences in approach between therapists occur over the relevance of macro-political influences, such as cultural and institutional discourses, over the micro-dynamics of therapeutic dialogue, as the focus of therapy (Monk & Gehart, 2003). One finds similar differences in discursive forms of research where the focus can be macro, as in the case of critical discourse analysis, or micro, as in the case of conversational analysis (Gale, Lawless, & Roulston, 2004). Regardless, the focus of discursive therapists is to converse with help clients change their problem-sustaining or problem-saturated discourse, be that from problem talk to solution talk, bad to better stories, or hosting collaborative dialogues focused on client preference and resourcefulness (Friedman, 1993). Thus, discursive therapists have been particularly interested in conversational practices helpful in deconstructing problem meanings while co-constructing more client-preferred meanings and directions (Paré, 2013).

While discursive therapists (Lock & Strong, 2012) borrow from discourse theory, their models do so quite differently. Narrative therapists (White & Epston, 1990; White, 2007), for example, draw heavily from Foucault, using questions to externalize and make explicit the workings of dominant discourses and stories in clients' lives, so that clients can consider and possibly enact more preferred alternatives. Solution-focused therapists (e.g., deShazer, 1994) negotiate clients' ways of talking/understanding from problem-focused language games to solution-focused, strengths-informed language games. Collaborative therapists (Anderson, 1997) see conversation as the means by which problems organize people's thinking and interacting, needed are pragmatic conversations that dissolve the problem-organized conversations, so that more preferred conversations can occur. Reflexive questions as conversational interventions are central to these meaning-focused therapies (Tomm, 1987); that is, questions are used intentionally, to invite from clients deconstructive conversations associated with problem meaning, or to invite conversations that construct preferred meanings, such as solutions. Common across these discursive therapies is a socially constructed view that meaning is revisable, though not correctly knowable in some general way. It would be wrong, however, to regard discursive therapies as only those just described. Increasingly, therapist-researchers are attending to emergent meanings in therapy, focusing on "responsiveness," pointing to a reflexive or discursive dimension of an otherwise normally practiced therapy (Kramer & Stiles, 2015).

Discourse analysts have largely approached psychotherapy critically, as a suspect institutional activity focused on "helping" clients adjust to normative societal expectations. This line of critique has been most evident in the "psy-complex" program of research of Nikolas Rose (1985) and influenced by Foucault's writing on discourse and "biopower" (1962, 2006). While discursive therapists have often had backgrounds in psychology, these discursive researchers more typically have brought a sociological focus to their examinations of therapy. Family therapy has been somewhat unique for owing some of its origins to communicationally focused research at the Mental Research Institute in Palo Alto, California (e.g., Watzlawick, Bevan Bavelas, & Jackson, 1967). A common sociological derivation for many discourse analysts is Garfinkel's (1967) ethnomethodological studies where the focus is on social orders and their tacit performance in socially situated, yet accountable ways. This focus more specifically tends to be on the micro-interactional features of therapeutic discourse as they occur between client and therapist moment-by-moment, turn by conversational turn. Most commonly, this focus is associated with conversation analysis (e.g., Peräkylã, Antaki, Vehviläinen, & Leudar, 2008), and rarely is it found in mainstream therapy research journals. More often, such studies appear in sociology and discourse analysis journals. Regardless of the kind of discursive research done of therapeutic discourse, very little of it currently influences the practice of discursive therapy.

Perhaps this psychological/sociological divide can help to explain why discursive therapists and discursive researchers are working apart. Psychology has tended to focus on individual behaviors, cognitions, and emotions largely bracketing off social influences, whereas sociology turns to cultural, institutional, and social influences when accounting for the same things psychologists attribute to the individual. In some respects, discourse or language use complicates things further, cutting across both individuals and social entities. People's words are not determined socially, even in face-to-face encounters Goffman (1967) saw as being "where the action is," though socially derived "involvement obligations" may influence what gets said. Individuals, as phenomenology has shown, bring their subjectivities to such conversations, and that means differences in their interpretive histories, habits, and preferences. Such differences can make for interesting conversational interactions, particularly in therapy. Whether one refers to such interactions as micro-social or inter-subjective, there is much worth studying as clients and therapists use discourse to transcend differences and make differences in clients' lives.

Critical discourse analysts have helped to expose the professional conversations of therapists with clients, as sites of societal reproduction (Rose, 1990). A related and derogatory term from a few decades ago was that therapists were "reality adjusters." This can seem a heavy-handed critique for therapists steeped in the understandings and aims of the human potential movement. For them, therapy aimed to be liberating, a means to optimizing oneself and becoming more real. Concerns about institutionalized "therapy" go back decades, as movies like "The Snake Pit" (Litvak, 1948) or "One Flew Over the Cuckoo's Nest" (Forman, 1975) attest. Concern about "treatment" for "mental health concerns" also focused Michel Foucault's PhD thesis, published in a revised form as "Madness and Civilization" (1962). How the concerns of therapy's prospective clientele are represented in discourses is part of the critical discourse analysts' concern (e.g., Parker, Georgaca, Harper, McLaughlin, & Stowell-Smith, 1996). Therapy, having many of its roots in psychology, tends to locate such concerns inside the psyches of clients who need therapists' services to correct or direct clients according to their models of practice. This discursive focus on inner life obscures the potential of outer injustices and distress to be seen and addressed as legitimate targets of intervention. Another concern has been with the way that therapeutic and psychological discourse has come to inform attempts to socially engineer our public and private institutions, professions, and ways of life (e.g., House, 2004; Miller & Rose, 2008). The key issue is with dominant discourses, especially for how they dominate our thinking and conversing, while displacing other discursive alternatives.

A Discursive Divide Between Research and Therapy?

Readers might wonder: why are discursive therapists and discursive researchers not reaching and influencing each other more? Surely discursive therapists who take socially constructive meaning making as a primary premise would be interested in what researchers who share their premise and study what such meaning making involves. In our experiences of trying to straddle this divide, we have found opinions on both sides frustrating at times. Discourse analysts, who strive to make their analytic process and claims transparent, transcribe actual talk to a level of detail that is exacting, to show how particular discursive interactions occurred, and to link analysis of those interactions to what was (and was not) produced in and from them. We have had colleagues and editors of therapy journal question why transcripts were necessary for supporting our analytic claims. Discursive researchers, for their part, can sometimes seem infatuated with Foucault, seeing every "therapeutic" turn at talk as coercing clients to take up institutionally expected discourse. Many discourse analysts, in other words, regard therapists as an institutional version of Garfinkel's (1967) "cultural dopes," implicitly serving institutional or ideological agendas they have not adequately reflected upon. Or worse, they subjugate clients into using the discourses of their preferred models of practice. Such misunderstandings suggest missed opportunities between discursive therapists and discursive researchers.

Our guess is that some of these caricatures of each other's work arise out of a distance that leads discursive therapists to dismiss discursive researchers, and vice versa. Most therapists are accustomed to reading *outcome* research, whereas discourse analysts focus more on discursive *processes*, particularly the language and meanings used in important interactions. Discourse for most therapy researchers and practitioners is uninteresting, save for how its use in conveying information or directives. Therapists tend to work from an information/reception model of communication (Turnbull, 2003) or from a speech-act (Searle, 1981) view, that their talk should yield responses in accordance with social norms and roles for the topic under discussion. Discourse analysts tend to be more dialogic and focused on responsive communications, while still focusing on how epistemic authority plays out in inquisitive pursuit of dominant therapist discourses and institutional agendas. Therapy can seem a dialogic contest where clients are inevitably the losers, by this view. In today's era of evidence-based therapy (e.g., Levant, 2005), the focus has largely been on "what works" and less on how what works (namely, interventions) can be shown to work through careful discursive analyses. By the information transmission/reception model of communication, interventions require precise communication to be delivered and received/acted upon as such. Little attention has been given to the not always straightforward conversational interactions where such important details as understanding, agreement, and next steps are worked out between therapist and client. The discourse analysts' attention to process, and what comes from it, is central to discursive research. Discursive researchers want to connect social and cultural interactions, including face-to-face turn-taking in dialogic interactions, to discourses used and to outcomes: to what gets produced from such dialogues or cultural conversations. When discursive therapists profess that they collaborate with clients in socially constructive dialogues, discursive researchers study such claims empirically.

Discursive Research of the Discursive Therapies?

Recently, Jerry Gale and Tom Strong (Strong & Gale, 2013) wrote about "postmodern clinical research," a phrase that some might read as an oxymoron. For many people, the social sciences seemed to go off the empirical rails in the postmodern/poststructuralist era. Part of the issue was over whether the structures identified, classified, and studied in the social sciences could be studied "as they were." Another part related to whether qualitative methods (like discourse analysis) had any business being part of social science at all; or, whether the outcomes of social science had any applicable value to questions of policy or practice. The philosophy of science imported from the natural sciences to inform social science research was one of linear causality, yet it seemed incapable of producing a psychological equivalent to physics' laws of gravity when it came to people and their interactions. The world humans live in is interpreted, refracted through the language and discourses we use, and that makes meaning important as it relates to human understanding and social behavior (Harré & Secord, 1972). We act from understandings of things, how things purportedly are does not usually direct our behavior, in Pavlovian fashion.

Much of qualitative research takes up this view, that participant accounts give us required insights into human action. Such accounts are not possible in performing human interactions, and talking about them afterwards can produce very different accounts from those provided by the participants in those interactions (Scott & Lyman, 1968). Phenomenologically speaking, people bring different ways of making sense to such meaning-making interactions, extending to what they take away from them. One line of discursive research comes from this recognition, that participants draw from different discourses or interpretive repertoires (Wetherell, 1998) when offering such accounts. In the popular media, such discourses are what so variably carve up the media streams that are informing and entertaining us. Consistent with Lyotard's (1984) pronouncement that postmodernity meant an end to metanarratives, discourse theorists, researchers, and therapists accept no neutral or objective "view from nowhere" (Nagel, 1989). They also are wary of any social consensus on how things are to be understood and acted upon, a post-modern view informing much of today's qualitative research (Denzin & Lincoln, 2017). The discursive researcher's curiosity is for how difference plays out in varied forms of human interaction and communication, though in this volume the focus is on therapeutic discourse.

Research of social interactions required a different methodological approach, one that could show how social interaction is performed, extending to what results in and from it. For newcomers to the relational ontology of this discursive approach (mostly CA, but also discursive psychology and some narrative research), a kind of vertigo can initially set in as inter-subjectivity becomes the focus when subjectivity has been the default ontology most people operate from. This is a dialogic ontology, Bakhtin's (1981) world developed from the in-between of people responding to each other, though much more is entailed than mere information transfers and receipts. People's interactions are not so linear and predictable, a pause or a gesture in the wrong place can disrupt people in the midst of their conversing, or invite a new passage of talk to work out, face-to-face, in how the speakers manage their responses to each other. This is a reflexive context where family therapists have acknowledged for decades (Watzlawick et al., 1967) that they cannot *not* communicate when they are face-to-face with clients. Instead, that same reflexive sense guides how discursively aware therapists (Strong, 2016) negotiate relationships, processes, and meanings through how they respond to clients turn by conversational turn. It is what gets used, done, and results from those negotiations that interest discursive researchers of the micro-persuasion. How do clients and therapists talk their way to a shared understanding, an agreed-to homework assignment, or a completed intervention?

For many therapists, research is a resource for becoming better at their work with clients. When it is good, it helps them recognize aspects of their work of which they had formerly been unaware, or it suggests new strategies, or improvements to existing strategies, they might effectively use. However, there are times when research seems turned against the frontline therapist or is used to micro-manage aspects of their practice. Such has sometimes been the case with the evidence-based movement in therapy, a movement largely imported from medicine, where highly specified protocols (or manuals) have been standardized and the therapist's job is to reliably reproduce them in interactions with clients (Timmermans & Berg, 2003). Partly in response to these concerns, a practice-based evidence movement has been recently developing (Green & Latchford, 2012; Prescott, Maeschalk, & Miller, 2017). This latter movement focuses on how therapists can learn from clients what it is that makes their work helpful, and to use that feedback to enhance their interactions with clients. There are few examples of using discursive research for such purposes, but Jerry Gale (2010) has been exploring its uses as a self-supervision resource for some time, to help therapists enhance their conversational practice. Discursive research tends not to answer the yes/no and how much kinds of questions therapists are accustomed to in the research literature. So, what might they gain from discursive research?

Discourse can seem an abstract construct to begin with, particularly when referring to therapeutic communication as discourse. Our personal journey into discursive research came because we wanted to explore what occurs within socially constructive dialogues, like those presented in the discursive therapy books of the 1990s. There one found crisp therapist utterances, artful questions, and clients responding in ways consistent with the practitioner-author's model of practice. Our experience of such communications was that they were messier. Still, the discursive ideas in these books drew our attention to features of therapeutic dialogue we had been taking for granted. How do discourses feature in the communications of therapists and clients was one such curiosity. An equally perplexing challenge was inter-subjectivity implied as it relates to therapeutic communications. How does understanding occur, and what does it mean to be understood, for example? Discursive answers to these kinds of questions can seem to defy clinical and common sense. Does it matter that a client speaks in a discourse different from that of her therapist, or why do these conversation analysts belabor the significance of a three-second pause before a therapist responds to a client? What became clearer with time for us was that discursive research could help attune therapists to therapeutic communication's hows and whats—and yes, it could help expose therapist dominance despite their claims to be collaborative.

Discursive Therapists and Discursive Researchers in This Book

The authors brought together for this edited volume approach therapy and discursive research of therapy from varied theoretical and methodological perspectives. The book aims to get therapists and researchers, who share a discursive perspective, reading and learning from each other. Therapists, relatively new to discursive research, should gain an appreciation for what motivates discourse analysts to look at their work. Why is it that discourse analysts focus so exactingly on words, how those words are used, and what comes from that use in therapy? Researchers, in turn, will learn from our therapist authors' conversational practices associated with a discursively informed therapy. Surely, therapists must recognize their complicity in holding clients to an unjust societal status quo, or what is it about the conversational work of therapy that so-focuses these well-intended therapists? Our hope is to facilitate new dialogues and potential lines of research that enhance therapeutic practice on discursive terms.

We (Olga and Tom) are both therapists who took a discursive turn—into doing therapy, and researching it. Interested in both the micro- and macro-approaches to discourse, as a focus in therapy and in our research, our many conversations have circled around two primary tensions associated with discursive research and practice. The first is a concern we think should pre-occupy any therapist: what possible good can come from a single therapist and client talking together, when power and wellbeing across the world are so unequally distributed? Why see therapy as a means to help clients find a voice in therapy, when they cannot use that voice beyond therapy? Are therapists not deluding themselves when they think their questions and conversationally shared interventions can make differences when the social and institutional structures in clients' lives are already so overdetermined? And what about therapist privilege and power when it comes to clients' interactions with them? Such questions can come up, particularly from sociologically oriented researchers and therapists for whom therapy might be a minor personal salve on gaping societal wounds. The flip-side concern relates why we think discursive therapy might make a difference in clients' lives. Does helping clients become more discursively aware and resourceful (Strong, 2016) through therapeutic dialogue translate beyond counselling? What makes for good therapy in clients' eyes, and how can discourse analysis better orient therapists to recognizing and enacting what does make a difference? Can therapists still be helpful in small-picture ways, recognizing that larger societal influences will remain the same? Such macro- and micro-concerns and questions about therapy, and discursive research of therapy animate discussions, case examples, and passages of therapy, throughout this volume.

Following this opening chapter, we shift to Jarl Wahlström review of therapeutic consultations at a Finnish university training center. Using a two-step procedure, his focus was to identify the words used to "create" therapeutic practice between therapist and client, drawing on Wampold's contextual model to delineate three discursive pathways for dialogue. Discursive differences are evident in what therapists and clients say, differences that cue up distinct therapeutic practices based on whether the words used predominantly are medical, psychological, or colloquial (i.e., lay) terms. The psychological discourse, in particular, shows therapists and clients co-constructing an inner mind to work on through their conversational work.

Subjectivity itself is often a focus of therapeutic discourse, and Evrinomy Avdi and Eugenie Georgaca examine subjectivity discourse in the context of a Greek couple's therapy. This presents a natural paradox in that relationships are inter-subjective contexts where subjectivity discourse aims to articulate individual experiences and preferences but in ways that do not alienate or disqualify partners. Drawing from social constructionist and discourse positioning theory, they examine how partners in a couple "position" their subjective experience and intentions, as well as each other's experience, as does their therapist. The analyses draw attention to how such accounts of subjectivity are "called upon" or proactively demonstrated. Given how much stock therapists tend to place in conversing from clients' subjective utterances, this chapter may give some pause with respect to the role that discourse plays in subjectivity talk.

A recurring finding in the psychotherapy research literature has been that clients' evaluation of the therapeutic alliance with their therapist is central to good therapy. Adam Horvath (1994) has been a key influence on this literature as the developer of the frequently used Working Alliance Inventory. However, such self-report instruments rely on retrospective evaluations of therapeutic interactions. In this chapter, Horvath along with Peter Muntigl uses conversation analysis to examine how the Working Alliance is *performed* conversationally in a therapeutic consultation by the famous family therapist, Salvador Minuchin. Their analysis, which includes attention to the nonverbal components of Minuchin's interactions with clients, helps to draw attention to actions most commonly evaluated as therapist attributes or qualities.

Gale Miller examines the practice of the discursive therapies through the analytic lens of ethnographies of institutional discourse. A sociologist and longtime contributor to solution-focused therapy, Miller here uses ethnomethodological, conversation analysis and Foucauldian discourse analyses lenses to examine the claims of collaborative practice advocated by discursive therapists for the immediacies of their dialogues with clients. The analyses of these micro-views of discursive therapy practice, in larger institutional context, draw needed critical attention to the macro-influences at work in dialogues intended to be collaborative and generative.

Given a longstanding emphasis on therapist objectivity, it has been only recently that the reflexive potentials of asking questions have become a focus of therapist authors. Questions are not neutral data-gathering instruments, they can be seen as conversational interventions in their own right. The potentials of questions as interventions, articulated by Karl Tomm (1987), have become a central feature of the conversational practices developed in narrative and solution-focused therapy. Joaquin Gaeta Silva, Olga Smoliak, and Shari Couture, who have worked with Tomm, explore therapists' questions as reflexive interventions in therapeutic dialogues, focusing specifically and empirically on what they construct in interactions between therapist and clients.

Drawing on social constructionist and critical discourse ideas pertaining to gendered power relations in therapy, Carmen Knudson-Martin with therapist-researchers have been developing a new discursive approach: Socio-Emotional Relationship Therapy (or SERT). In their chapter, they describe how they brought together an action-research focus with grounded theory and narrative forms of analysis, to identify discourses and discourse positions that can serve as the target of intervention in relational therapy. For readers interested in how gendered power relations become evident in relational therapy, and how discursive therapists can respond, the chapter provides insight into how micro- and macro-politics associated with discourse can be assessed and addressed in discursive approaches to therapy.

Practicing therapy discursively calls for some added ethical sensitivities and sensibilities beyond those normally associated with professional practice. Specifically, discursive therapists focus on the deconstructive and constructive potentials of language use in dialogue, and as they do, they need to attend to their own potentials to dominate the meaning making of discursive therapy. There are both macro- and micro-influences to consider, some raised in earlier chapters, but where such influences play out is in the responsive face-to-face communications of therapists and clients. Strong and Smoliak focus on zooming in and out on the roles, institutional and cultural discourses, and the negotiation of meaning and conversational process ostensibly occurring between clients and therapists. They do so by considering notions like professional authority, the use of questions, evidence-informed practice, and social justice—as such notions feature in Keeney's (1983) aesthetic view of therapist-client dialogues.

A premise of this book is that discursive research of discursive therapy is still in its early stages. If the discursive therapist's claim is that conversations with clients provide opportunities to reflect upon taken-for-granted meaning and generate alternative meanings, how can this be shown to occur? Eleftheria Tseliou provides a big picture overview of ways discursive research can be used to study psychotherapy processes and outcomes derived from those processes. She surveys contrasting ideas and methods used in discursive approaches to therapy process research, bringing a well-trained eye for how these methods may be helpful to therapist-researchers curious about the "here and now" of clinical work.

The book closes with the critical reflections of renowned psychotherapy process researcher, Bill Stiles, regarding the potentials of researching therapy on discursive terms. This concluding chapter speaks to researchers and therapists who want to take a discursive approach further in supplementing their understandings and practice of therapy. Given the primary focus of psychotherapy research on outcomes, Stiles' longstanding focus on the links between therapy processes and potential outcomes offers readers expanded ways to relate to the conversational or discursive work of therapy.

Coda

Our interest in this volume is in bringing together two professional communities—therapists who practice in discursive ways and discursive researchers—in ways that such community members might learn and benefit from each other's work. Both communities developed out of a dissatisfaction with how discourse and meaning could be relevant to the conversational work of psychotherapy. Both communities were dissatisfied with metaphors of language use that obscured how meaning occurred in (or was constrained by) communicative interaction. If therapy is a talking "cure," why not take seriously how clients and therapists talk and listen to each other, to research what their talking and listening is doing, and has purported capacities to change? The big concern of early discursive therapists was with how conventional research was used to discredit their work; indeed, that unconventionality seemed part of the allure in those early days. However, therapists weren't the only professionals then talking about discourses, stories, and transformative rhetoric. Discursive researchers developed their work in related ways, yet in an almost parallel universe, where only rarely would there be useful interchanges with discursive therapists. We think there have been too many missed opportunities, and so we have invited the discursive therapists and discursive researchers in this volume to showcase their important discursive work.

References

Anderson, H. (1997). *Conversation, language, and possibilities*. New York, NY: Basic Books.

Bakhtin, M. (1981). *The dialogic imagination* (M. Holquist, Ed.; C. Emerson & M. Holquist, Trans.). Austin, TX: University of Texas Press.

Denzin, N., & Lincoln, Y. (Eds.). (2017). *The Sage handbook of qualitative research* (5th ed.). Los Angeles, CA: Sage.

deShazer, S. (1994). *When words were originally magic*. New York, NY: W. W. Norton.
Fanon, F. (1967). *Black skin, white masks* (C. Farrington, Trans.). New York, NY: Grove Press.
Forman, M. (1975). *One flew over the cuckoo's nest*. Fantasy films. S. Zaentz & M. Douglas, Producers.
Foucault, M. (1962). *Madness & civilization* (R. Howard, Trans.). New York, NY: Vintage.
Foucault, M. (1973). *The order of things: An archaeology of the human sciences* (A. M. Sheridan Smith, Trans.). New York, NY: Vintage.
Foucault, M. (2006). *Psychiatric power: Lectures at the College de France 1973–1974* (J. LaGrange, Ed.; G. Burchill, Trans.). New York, NY: Palgrave Macmillan.
Frances, A. (2013). *Saving normal*. New York, NY: Wm. Morrow.
Friedman, S. (Ed.). (1993). *The new language of change*. New York, NY: Guilford.
Gadamer, H.-G. (1988). *Truth and method* (2nd ed.; J. Weinsheimer & D. G. Marshall, Trans.). New York, NY: Continuum.
Gale, J. (2010). Discursive analysis: A research approach for studying the moment-to-moment construction of meaning in systemic practice. *Human Systems: The Journal of Therapy, Consultation & Training, 21*(2), 7–37.
Gale, J., Lawless, J., & Roulston, K. (2004). Discursive approaches to clinical research. In T. Strong & D. Paré (Eds.), *Furthering talk: Advances in the discursive therapies* (pp. 125–144). New York: Kluwer Academic/Plenum Press.
Garfinkel, H. (1967). *Studies in ethnomethodology*. Englewood Cliffs, NJ: Prentice Hall.
Goffman, E. (1967). *Interaction ritual: Essays on face-to-face behavior*. New York, NY: Pantheon.
Green, D., & Latchford, G. (2012). *Maximising the benefits of psychotherapy: A practice-based evidence approach*. West Sussex, UK: Wiley-Blackwell.
Harré, R., & Secord, P. (1972). *The explanation of social behaviour*. Oxford, UK: Basil Blackwell.
Horvath, A. O. (1994). Research on the alliance. In A. O. Horvath & L. S. Greenberg (Eds.), *The working alliance: Theory, research and practice* (pp. 259–285). New York, NY: John Wiley & Sons.
House, R. (2004). *Therapy beyond modernity*. London, UK: Karnac.
Illouz, E. (2008). *Saving the modern soul: Therapy, emotions, and the culture of self-help*. Berkeley, CA: University of California Press.
Keeney, B. P. (1983). *Aesthetics of change*. New York, NY: Guilford.

Kramer, U., & Stiles, W. B. (2015). The responsiveness problem in psychotherapy: A review of proposed solutions. *Clinical Psychology: Science and Practice, 22*, 277–295.
Levant, R. F. (2005). *Report of the 2005 presidential task force on evidence-based practice*. American Psychological Association. Retrieved from https://www.apa.org/practice/resources/evidence/evidence-based-report.pdf
Litvak, A. (1948). *The snake pit*. Film Produced by 20th Century Fox.
Lock, A. J., & Strong, T. (Eds.). (2012). *Discursive perspectives on therapeutic practice*. New York, NY: Oxford University Press.
Lyotard, J.-F. (1984). *The postmodern condition: A report on knowledge* (G. Bennington & B. Massumi, Trans.). Minneapolis, MN: University of Minnesota Press.
McNamee, S., & Gergen, K. J. (Eds.). (1992). *Therapy as social construction*. Newbury Park, CA: Sage.
Miller, P., & Rose, N. (Eds.). (2008). *Governing the present*. Cambridge, UK: Polity.
Monk, G., & Gehart, D. R. (2003). Sociopolitical activist or conversational partner? Distinguishing the position of the therapist in narrative and collaborative therapies. *Family Process, 42*(1), 19–30.
Nagel, T. (1989). *The view from nowhere*. New York, NY: Oxford University Press.
Ortega, F., & Vidal, F. (Eds.). (2011). *Neurocultures: Glimpses into an expanding universe*. Frankfurt am Main, Germany: Peter Lang.
Paré, D. (2013). *The practice of collaborative counseling and psychotherapy: Developing skills in culturally mindful helping*. Los Angeles, CA: Sage.
Parker, I., Georgaca, E., Harper, D., McLaughlin, T., & Stowell-Smith, M. (Eds.). (1996). *Deconstructing psychopathology*. London, UK: Sage.
Pepper, S. C. (1942). *World hypotheses: A study of evidence*. Berkeley, CA: University of California Press.
Peräkylã, A., Antaki, C., Vehviläinen, S., & Leudar, I. (Eds.). (2008). *Conversation analysis and psychotherapy*. Cambridge, UK: Cambridge University Press.
Prescott, D. S., Maeschalk, C. L., & Miller, S. D. (Eds.). (2017). *Feedback-informed treatment in clinical practice: Reaching for excellence*. Washington, DC: American Psychological Association.
Rose, N. (1985). *The psychological complex: Psychology, politics and society in England, 1869–1939*. London, UK: Routledge & Kegan Paul.
Rose, N. (1990). *Governing the soul*. New York, NY: Routledge.
Scott, M. B., & Lyman, S. M. (1968). Accounts. *American Sociological Review, 33*(1), 46–62.

Searle, J. R. (1981). *Speech acts: An essay in the philosophy of language*. New York, NY: Cambridge University Press.

Strong, T. (2016). Discursive awareness and resourcefulness: Bringing discursive researchers into closer dialogue with discursive therapists? In M. O'Reilly & J. Lester (Eds.), *The Palgrave handbook of adult mental health: Discourse and conversation studies* (pp. 481–501). London, UK: Palgrave Macmillan.

Strong, T., & Gale, J. (2013). Postmodern clinical research: In and out of the margins. *Journal of Systemic Therapies, 32*(2), 46–57.

Timmermans, S., & Berg, M. (2003). *The gold standard: The challenge of evidence-based medicine and standardization in health care*. Philadelphia, PA: Temple University Press.

Tomm, K. (1987). Interventive interviewing: Part II. Reflexive questioning as a means to enable self-healing. *Family Process, 26*, 167–183.

Turnbull, W. (2003). *Language in action: Psychological models of conversation*. New York, NY: Psychology Press.

Watzlawick, P., Bevan Bavelas, J., & Jackson, D. D. (1967). *Pragmatics of human communication*. New York, NY: W. W. Norton.

Weisstein, N. (1971). Psychology constructs the female; or the fantasy life of the male psychologist (with some attention to the fantasies of his friends, the male biologist and the male anthropologist). *Social Education, 35*, 362–373.

Wetherell, M. (1998). Positioning and interpretative repertoires: Conversation analysis and post-structuralism in dialogue. *Discourse & Society, 9*, 387–412.

White, M. (2007). *Maps of narrative practice*. New York, NY: W. W. Norton.

White, M., & Epston, D. (1990). *Narrative means to therapeutic ends*. New York, NY: W. W. Norton.

Wittgenstein, L. (1953). *Philosophical investigations* (G. E. M. Anscombe, Trans.). Oxford, UK: Blackwell.

2

Discourse in Psychotherapy: Using Words to Create Therapeutic Practice

Jarl Wahlström

Bruce E. Wampold (2001; Wampold & Imel, 2015) has, based on systematic reviews of meta-analyses of randomized, controlled clinical trials, made a strong case against what he calls *the medical model* of how psychotherapy works. That model would imply that the remedial effect of psychotherapy would be founded on the prescribed use of some appropriate therapeutic technique, targeted at some specific disorder of mental health. But, says Wampold, findings from decades of quantitative outcome research do not fit this meta-model. He argues for the adoption of an alternative meta-model, *the contextual model*, when trying to grasp how psychotherapy works.

The contextual model outlines three basic pathways through which the effect of psychotherapy is achieved (Wampold & Imel, 2015). The first pathway is the real personal relationship between client and therapist which, based on trust, creates a social connection and a sense of belonging. The second pathway is the expectation of client and therapist alike that the specific form of therapy they are engaging in will have beneficial

J. Wahlström (✉)
Department of Psychology, University of Jyväskylä, Jyväskylä, Finland
e-mail: jarl.wahlstrom@jyu.fi

O. Smoliak, T. Strong (eds.), *Therapy as Discourse*, The Language of Mental Health,
https://doi.org/10.1007/978-3-319-93067-1_2

effects. The third pathway constitutes the concrete therapeutic actions—in sessions, as well as in other life situations—the client gets involved in during the process. What this meta-model emphasizes, in contrast to the medical model, is the nature of psychotherapy as *social practice*.

Wampold's (2001) contextual model suggests the importance of looking at how the social practice of psychotherapy is actually *done*. How is the practice of psychotherapy, as a specialized social institution, designed to deal with peoples' experiences of lost mastery in their lives, established through the mutual conversational actions of the client and the therapist? The aim of this chapter is to propose one approach to that question. Applying a data corpus of actual initial therapy sessions, I will look at how clients use different discursive resources, that is, means to express oneself afforded by the rich variety of possible language uses, to present themselves in their first interview as prospective consumers of therapy; how therapists respond to this in various ways; how clients and therapists jointly build agendas of relevant topics; and how these themes are discussed adopting linguistic resources from three different social discourses.

Approaching Psychotherapy as Social Practice

The most fundamental tenets of the discursive approach, as applied in this chapter, are that language is not only a device for depicting reality and that the social world is constructed through the uses of varieties of institutionalized forms of speech. Charles Taylor (2016) refers to this duality as the designative and constitutive functions of language. Different terms, such as speech genres, language games, linguistic registers, repertoires, and discourses, are used in the literature to refer to the constitutive forms of language. Using different forms of speech, actors—as interlocutors in conversations—create conversational contexts, adopt positions in interaction, initiate meaning systems, and open and close different possible action lines.

Two excerpts from the conversation between a therapist Tarja and her client Eija demonstrate this:

Eija: and then insufficiency of the thyroid gland may cause all these ((symptoms))

Tarja: *perhaps it was then there as some kind of*

Eija: yes, and now they have noticed hypertension and it's being medicated

Tarja: *and do you also have medication for the thyroid insufficiency*

Eija; yes, I have

Tarja: *so it is now being treated*

In her responses Tarja acknowledged Eija's somatic complaints but by saying "it is now being treated" marked them as being outside the realm of psychotherapy. Then again, in the following extract, Tarja made a point of the difference between visible appearance and inner experience:

Tarja: *well, I don't know if anybody has told you and how you talk but one doesn't notice in you that inner experience that* [yeah], *I wouldn't guess from your appearance that you are anxious* [mm] *but it is often* [mm] *or usually it is more like an inner* [mm] *feeling, more an inner feeling of anxiousness in that situation.*

Tarja's turn fashioned an image of the phenomena of mind as private and not necessarily easily observed, and, hence, worth of exploring in psychotherapy. Such instances of language use specify the social context and the respective roles and positions of the two interlocutors as client and therapist. Then, to successfully perform the practice of "doing psychotherapy," the participants—clients and therapists—need to subscribe to particular *social discourses* (Harper, 2006; Potter, 2003). The goal of the present chapter is to identify and describe at least some of those discourses.

The term discourse may be used in at least two different meanings (Wiggins, 2017). First to refer to a progressive, dynamic, and social process where meanings are produced and modified. Discourse in this sense is synonymous to the term *conversation*, the word which will be used in this chapter when referring to the concrete social process of discourse. Second, as mentioned above, the term discourse is used to refer to an institutionalized variety of language use, which can be identified based on choices of vocabulary, key metaphors, grammatical constructions, and so on. As such, discourses act as resources and restrictions for what can be said and meant, and who can say and give meaning in different situations, and from various positions (Avdi & Georgaca, 2007). In this chapter, the term discourse will be used in this sense.

The discursive perspective emphasizes that *meanings* are produced and co-constructed in conversation, through an interplay of *text* (i.e. what is said or written in natural language, or displayed by some other form of semiotic system) and *context* (the situation, the circumstances, and the relational field) (Wahlström, 2006). Contexts are not given or predefined, they are created, evoked, and negotiated by the interlocutors in conversational action. The uses of different discourses, however, shape conversational practices and induce various meaning systems. In these systems the meaning of words and terms appear as given and fixed. A typical example is the use of diagnostic categories in medical discourse; for example, "depression" has apparently one single meaning, shared by all participants—and thus the constructed quality and negotiability of the term goes unnoticed. Challenging such fixed meanings requires a change of the discourse adopted by the interlocutors in the conversation.

A Data Corpus of Psychotherapy Talk

In this chapter, I will show instances of language uses in a natural setting of psychotherapy sessions. I use a data corpus from the first sessions of nine psychotherapies, conducted by five therapists, that took place at a university training clinic in Finland. Four of the therapists (all female), whom I have given the pseudonyms Tanja, Tarja, Tea, and Tuula, were licensed psychologists, with at least two years of clinical practice (but usually more), who participated in a specialization program in integrative psychotherapy. One therapist, Tero, was an experienced male psychotherapy trainer, who was conducting the session with one female trainee, Tiina, as co-therapist. Eight of the clients, here called Anna, Arja, Eija, Helena, Laura, Mari, Miina, and Susanna, were female, and one, Risto, male. The age range of the clients was from 19 to 45. They were all self-referred and their presenting problems, as reported in their first phone call when booking the session, included depression, fatigue, social anxiety, stress, panic attacks, coping with divorce, and binging and purging.

The sessions were conducted in Finnish. Videotaping and the use of the sessions for research purposes took place with the informed and documented consent of clients and therapists. For this chapter extracts from the original complete verbatim transcriptions[1] of the recordings were translated into English. When translating I have made an effort to preserve the original style, grammatical composition, and vocabulary use of the original as much as possible, while at the same time make the extracts accessible and comprehensible for the reader. No special symbols indicating prosody of speech or interactional features are included, since these were not the focus of interest.

Topical Themes and Discourses

When reading the original data, I followed a micro-analytic, data-driven "bottom-up" form of doing discourse analysis (Wiggins, 2017). This entailed two steps. The first one was answering the What-question, finding the *topical themes* of the conversations, that is, what was talked about in the discussions. The themes were identified using conventions of qualitative content analysis (Mayring, 2014). The second step was answering the How-question, finding the *forms of speech* in use, that is, the different discourses emerging from the data. The What- and How-questions consider respectively the two concurrent functions of language—the designative and the constitutive—as described by Taylor (2016), and are approached related to each other in the review of the findings.

When trying to identify different discourses, I mainly looked at the use of words and ways of expression, but also on topics, meaning systems, and functions. The notion of discourses as means of constructing particular social practices served as a basic guiding principle: could this particular form of speech be applicable in a variety of situations or does it appear to be restricted to and define a specific social practice?

[1] I acknowledge with thanks the contribution of Heidi Toivonen, M.A., who undertook the transcription work.

Six core topical themes that all therapist-client dyads covered in the first session could be identified:

- wording the problematic experience of the client and establishing a focus and a common ground for the therapeutic work;
- defining or commenting on the interactional context and the relation between the participants;
- working on a shared understanding of the reasons for the clients presenting problems;
- constructing the client's mind as an object of investigation;
- negotiating goals and tasks for the therapeutic work;
- constructing reformulations of the client's problems.

Three different discourses, clearly distinguishable from each other, could be identified:

- the *medical discourse* contained the use of professional psychiatric or other medical terms, mainly diagnostic labels ("since puberty I have had this kind of, … I don't know, is it a panic disorder or what is it"), and of similarly professional expressions using terminology from clinical psychology; the discourse was used to define and describe the presenting problem, earlier treatments, and present treatment arrangements;
- the *colloquial discourse* contained the use of ordinary language, common words and expressions, and sometimes quite individual or private metaphorical phrases ("every evening when I go to these AA groups, and there are new people present, …, so damn it, already four or five turns before my own, so hell how, when my turn approaches, I freeze"); the discourse was used to give descriptions of the client's problematic behavior and experiences; of his/her background, historical contexts, present social relationships, and contexts (family, working life); of his/her sensations, feelings, or conditions; of attitudes and characteristics of the client or significant others; and of treatment expectations and goals;
- the *therapeutic discourse* contained words and phrases referring to specific psychological realms of cognition, emotions, and experiencing

("so I do know that I am ill and like this but at the moment you binge you don't grasp that, it comes only after the binging and vomiting, it arises such a feeling of victory"); the discourse was used to inspect various phenomena of the mind, such as action patterns, thoughts, intentions, attributions; to formulate, validate, and interpret sensations, feelings, and experiences; to explore contexts, life situation, and social relations, either as sources of problems or as resources for relief; and to focus on the goal of treatment, treatment history, therapeutic situation and relation, and motivation.

The Use of Discourses When Discussing Different Topics

The colloquial and therapeutic discourses were used in all thematic areas but the medical discourse only in the first and third ones. The therapeutic discourse was most typically used in the second, fourth, and sixth area.

Talking About the Problematic Experience

When presenting their problems and painful experiences, clients sometimes used the medical discourse as a means to communicate to their therapists their reasons to seek help. Much more, however, they used common language and colloquial expressions to give an account of their concerns. These could be dramatic, colorful small stories or items of uncertain searching for appropriate expressions. The clients described their reasons for seeking help in colloquial terms of distressing feelings and problematic experiences, resulting in a sensation of lost mastery in some realm of life. The clients' accounts were usually responded to by the therapist in the same colloquial style, only in a few instances therapists took the initiative to use medical language. These features gave the impression that participants did not, as a rule, treat the situation only, or even primarily, as a formal professional encounter (as one might treat a visit to a medical doctor), but as an instance of forming a more personal relationship.

The description of the problematic experience took in many instances the form of mini-narratives from the clients' lives. For example, Arja, a 45-year-old school teacher, told one to her therapist Tuula[2]:

> Arja: when autumn was coming closer I understood that I can't in any way handle it [*just so, yeah*] and then I went to my workplace and I gathered all my stuff away and slammed the door behind me and decided that I will never return there anymore

Here Arja, wording her story in a colloquial fashion, gives a dramatic account of her difficulties. She, on one hand, tells about her inability to go on working, but then, on the other hand, presents herself as taking an agentic position when facing the situation—she "understands" her situation and makes an intentional decision "never to return." Even though she had earlier been given a diagnosis of bipolar disorder, and had a long "career" as a patient within the mental health services, when giving Tuula her reasons for seeking psychotherapy at the university clinic, she used most of the time to tell about her disappointments with her earlier treatments. She did mention her illness but used ordinary and expressive language when referring to her manic states:

> Arja: I got antidepressants and then it went over [*yeah*] towards the other end so that the reel started to roll too fast and it started to go too fast, and then the antidepressants had [*ok, yeah*] to be withdrawn in a hurry

She did not present the illness in itself as the most pressing issue:

> Arja: I have thought that it is my whole process that is in question, that this is no typical case of work burnout [*mm*], firstly I have this illness ((bipolar disorder)) and then secondly this surely is this kind of total problem [*mm*] of how to cope with life

[2] In the extracts, the client's speech is given in normal font, the therapist's speech is italicized. Small responses are shown within square brackets. Explanative additions are given within double rounded brackets. Deleted text is shown as three periods within square brackets.

Here, as was common in almost all cases, Arja uses vocabularies, for example, labels of some psychiatric diagnostic categories, from the medical discourse. In most cases these were, as in the example above, only briefly mentioned, and they were not much deliberated on as grounds for seeking help. Arja makes it explicit that she is not seeking remedy from any medical condition but, using a phrase typical for the therapeutic discourse, asking for help to tackle a more fundamental problem, "how to cope with life."

In a similar vein, Helena, a 35-year-old psychiatric nurse who in her initial telephone call had referred to her depression, in the actual meeting with Tuula, her therapist, used descriptive and experiential colloquial language:

> Helena: why I am here, is the feeling that now I cannot go forward anymore on my own, I am like grinding over and over again, the thoughts are kind of circling around the same track

Helena's description of her experience of vanished mastery in her life, her sense of lost agency, is vivid and detailed. The description actually entails two elements, a portrayal of her dysfunctional psychology ("grinding over and over again") and a statement on her situation ("I cannot go forward on my own"). Discursively the work done here is twofold—giving a reason for seeking psychological help and presenting the speaker as someone ready to work on her problems together with the therapist. Helena's turn serves to establish a common ground for the therapeutic work.

Eija, a 41-year-old special education teacher who in her initial telephone call had mentioned her fatigue and social anxiety as reasons for seeking therapy, actually in her talk with her therapist Tarja, used a lot of time to talk about her physical illnesses. In her responses Tarja, as shown earlier, acknowledged these somatic complaints but marked them as being outside the realm of psychotherapy. This was accentuated when she, in one of the very few instances this was done by the therapist, introduced a psychiatric diagnostic label as a means to redirect the conversation:

> Tarja: *and the social anxiety, you are a special education teacher, are* [yes] *you now* [yes], *you said that you are working and* [yes], *so is it especially in work that the anxiety comes forth*
> Eija: actually, it is in all contacts with adults

Tarja connects to the phone call and takes the diagnostic term "social anxiety" into use, thus delimiting the realm of the conversational context. This could be an indicator of the medical discourse but note that Tarja does not, however, treat the "social anxiety" as a predefined pathological entity (as one would in medical discourse) but, using the more generic form, "the anxiety" connects it to the social contexts of the client, in line with usages common to the therapeutic discourse. The use of a specific term does not as such determine which discourse is adopted. A similar cautious and conditional use of diagnostic labels can be seen also in the following data excerpt.

> Tarja: *yes, I try to get a better grip on your condition* [...] *you said* [...] *that it is more like fatigue* [...] *or is it more some kind of low spirits or depressive or does it involve some kind of hopelessness or how would you describe it*
> Eija: well I would call it fatigue, I'm not really hopeless, perhaps somewhat in low spirits, that is not a wrong word, but that kind [*yeah*] of depression I don't feel [*ok*], I am tired of all the aches and ailments [*yeah*], all of those things that I think are excessive in my life [*yeah*]

Again, unlike you would in medical discourse, Tarja's turn treats psychological phenomena such as "fatigue," "low spirits," and "hopelessness" as subjective, not very strictly defined and negotiable. These features, and the introduction "I try to get a better grip on your condition," are typical of the therapeutic discourse and distinguish this language use from the colloquial discourse. Tarja's turn serves to establish for her and Eija a common ground for their future collaboration. Eija, in her turn, adopts two positions—one as an observer of and authority on her condition and the other as a person ready to do something about "all those things" excessive in her life.

Talking About the Context and the Relation

Much of the discursive work clients and therapists do in their first encounter has to do with establishing the meeting as a shared context for conversation. This entails different tasks, one of them being defining the contact as a therapeutic relationship in making. This, although usually seen as a core professional function, could in the present data be done in quite informal ways. In all the dyads, there were some conversational exchange that commented on how the participants related to the situation and to their respective complementary roles and positions as client and therapist. The amount of this talk varied, however, a lot between the cases, and only some of the therapists made use of more formal therapeutic discourse when attempting to explicate issues relating to the therapeutic relationship.

For instance, Tuula, when talking to Helena about the importance of the therapeutic relationship, used colloquial and metaphorical language:

> Tuula: *these are terrible important also, let's say issues of personal chemistry* [mm] *or something like that, that you don't have to commit yourself without a trial period or somehow buy the pig in the sack, and of course everybody* ((different therapists)) *work in their own way*

Tuula uses the colloquial expressions "personal chemistry" and "buying the pig in the sack" when taking up two important aspects of establishing a therapeutic relationship—the mutual match or mismatch between the personal psychologies of the client and the therapist, and the entitlement of the client to make his/her own decision regarding whom to accept as the therapist to collaborate with. The use of colloquial discourse was in this example perhaps extreme, still it was the case that in most instances the therapists used colloquial expressions when talking about the therapy context, as if to avoid giving the appearance of a highly hierarchical professional relationship.

The clients could, in different ways, take the initiative to comment on the relationship. Arja, who had an experience of numerous psychological treatments extending over more than ten years, remarked on her difficulties in building a therapeutic relation in a way that resembled a professional use of therapeutic discourse:

Arja: somehow I think that earlier I had the view that I need the kind of therapist who is so intelligent that she twigs out when I am fooling her, but now I have I have realized that [*mm*] my problem anyway is on the emotional side so strongly that it does not really matter

Arja gives the impression of a client who is cognizant of her earlier inclination to put unilateral demands on her therapist and now, as if having learnt her lesson, understands that she has to admit that her own emotional problems are essential in shaping the relation. Such a presentation of oneself as both able and willing to enter the therapy in the position of a self-observant client was also given by Risto, a 45-year-old entrepreneur:

Risto: and then you ((looked at)) yourself, that still two and a half years ago my weight was one-hundred-and-fifteen kilos, and my bearing and everything, that like made you ((think)) no goddamn, and then a good friend of mine said what if we go there ((an AA group)) a little bit but that did not, I had myself in my own way to go through all those feelings, had to myself for my own sake and nobody else's seek ((help)) [*mm*] [...] and then two of my friends ((said)) like that, look a little bit at your childhood and your past, and then a self-examination like that

Risto constructs a story of himself as a person who, after more or less unfruitful encouragements from friends, finally has reached a proper inner motivation and insight in his need for help. He is now prepared to commence on a process of self-examination, an appropriate position for a prospective psychotherapy client.

In some instances, the interaction was talked about as an arena where clinically salient phenomena could be observed. Tarja and Eija discussed how her presenting problem of social anxiety was manifested in the therapy situation. Tarja responded to Eija's spontaneous expression with a rather elaborated piece of therapeutic discourse:

Eija: and of course, this is difficult that [*yeah*] you sit there and look [*yeah*] this way [*yeah, yes*] all the time

Tarja: *yeah, surely, do you have here also that kind of a feeling, that you mentioned before, that you have this feeling of shame, that you are being exposed, is it somehow present here in relation to the anxiety, like I said just before I cannot notice that in you*

Tarja introduces a sample of psychological theory where the feeling of anxiety is connected to another feeling, shame, and a cognitive notion of "being exposed." This is done, however, cautiously, in the form of a question, and with an allusion to the interactional setting—the therapist's observations do not correspond to the client's sensation. The reference to this incongruence serves as an invitation to further joint exploration.

Talking About the Reasons for the Problems

When exploring the possible reasons for the clients' present complaints and making connections to their life stories and present life situations, clients and therapists alike used a variety of discursive means, drawing upon linguistic resources from the medical, the colloquial, as well as the therapeutic discourse. There were no instances, though, where the therapist would attempt to give the client an "explanation" of his/her problem using resources from psychiatric or clinical discourse. Mostly the therapists attended to the clients' own ponderings on the reasons for their difficulties and occasionally supplemented them either following the clients form of speech, or introducing some interpretation or other comment from a therapeutic repertoire.

Quite commonly some characteristic or trait of the client was constructed as the "reason" for the problem at hand and that particular attribute was treated as an essential part of the client. For instance, using colloquial discourse, Tero and Mari, a 19-year-old high school pupil, constructed her "sensitivity" as such an essentialized reason for her problems:

> Tero: *yeah, yeah, you said something about you being in that way sensitive, sensitive to experience, yeah*
>
> Mari: yeah, I'm really sensitive in that way that I always take all things heavily

The impact of the client's family background on the client's present problems could be talked about in quite different ways. Risto started his session by giving, on his own initiative, Tea a long and detailed history of his life and difficulties, amounting to an almost professional exposition of the "etiology" of the condition, defined by himself as panic attacks:

> Risto: and, the childhood was always being on your guard, my father was anyway quite an alcoholic, and mother again was this type who was prone to depression, who dealt a lot with sedative medication, and then had four to five suicidal attempts which failed

In contrast to Risto's use of diagnostic labels and medical vocabulary, Laura, a 34-year-old high school teacher reporting burnout, depression, and social anxiety as her presenting problems, talking to Tarja, contemplated on her family background, and her own position in the relational field, in a more colloquial story-telling fashion:

> Laura: my elder sister was really bad at school, it was just a pain […] she has now made it good in life, but I remember somehow, they were not necessarily direct messages given to me but somehow so that I felt that something is expected from me

Although both accounts place the client and the history of his/her difficulties within the social matrix of family relations, there still is a decisive difference between them. In Risto's turn, drawing upon resources from the medical discourse, the diagnostic membership categories of the parents ("alcoholic," "depression") are offered as somehow self-evident and generic reasons for his later problems. In Laura's turn, again, the personal portrayal of her position in the family constellation affords a psychologically more vivid exposition, and hence a potential basis for constructing a shared observational position in the therapeutic conversational exchange.

In some instances, although not very often in these first sessions, the therapist suggested a connection between the family background and the present complaint. For example, Tuula, using therapeutic discourse, offered Helena a tentative explanation for her experience, and an alternative way of looking at her intentions.

> Tuula: *what is it then in your mother's phone calls that makes them so distressing, are they somehow especially distressing, you mother's calls*

Helena: well, when they are connected there to my birthplace and surely to those issues [*ok, yeah, yeah*], it then arises from there

Tuula: *have you somehow had this that you have wanted to detach yourself from these* ((issues)) *of your* [mm] *childhood family*

Tuula's question renders an earlier remark concerning her mother's phone calls by Helena as relevant for the conversation and worth of further exploration. Helena responds to this by making a connection between her present sentiments and her family history. This creates for Tuula an opportunity to suggest—in the form of a question—an intentional ground for Helena's stance in relation to the mother's calls. As such the question could pave the way for further meaning transforming conversational work.

Talking About the Client's Mind

A salient feature of therapeutic conversations is that "the mind" of the client, its operations and phenomena, becomes an object of observation and investigation. In the present data, this was accomplished mostly using conversational means from the therapeutic discourse, and on the initiative of the therapist. The responses given by the clients to these invitations varied and were mostly accomplished with means from the colloquial discourse. The different discursive efforts through which an image of the client's mind as a shared object for investigation was created served to afford the client a position from where to make observation on his/her own psychology. It appeared that this goal was more effectively achieved when the therapist joined the client's own linguistic register or showed affiliation with his/her emotional attitude, rather than if the therapist used elaborated expressions from the therapeutic discourse.

Tero, the seasoned therapist who was interviewing Mari, the high school girl who had reported social anxiety, was especially prone to formulate his questions so as to invite the respondent to look at the operations of her own mind:

Tero: *yeah, yeah, if you approach in your mind that situation so what, what were you afraid of, what was the emotion, what did it tell you*

Another discursive means was to give a tentative account of the mind's way of operating:

Mari: school is that kind of a place that is for me just like that which makes me feel terrible anxious

Tero: *yeah, yeah, so it's not only, quite like you feel that when you have daily to go to school then you in advance start to have such a reserved, protected, covered feeling*

These invitations, however, did not usually result in establishing a shared linguistic playground. For instance, when Tero invited Mari to look at her mind, Mari responded by talking about her immediate experiences:

Tero: *yeah, yeah, if you approach in your mind that situation so what, what were you afraid of, what was the emotion, what did it tell you*

Mari: well really that, I guess something that you can't control yourself, you just shake like that [*yeah*] and then you got scared of that [*mm*], I think that when I was in seventh grade I started to drink coffee and my body reacted really crazy to that [*the coffee, yeah*] so the shaking surely followed from that [*mm*] and then I just was frightened by that and I have feared that since then

Tero's elaborate use of the therapeutic discourse, formulating expressions like "approach your mind" or "what does the emotion tell," apparently did not resonate with Mari's concrete way of finding linguistic articulation of her experiences. Susanna, a 30-year-old doctoral student who had given her confusion with regard to her present life situation as reason to seek therapy, also gave a broad and evasive account of her life situation when responding to Tea's invitation to reflect on her thoughts in her mind:

Tea: *what were the thoughts that came to your mind when you started to think about them on your own*

> Susanna: well, something like, I don't know it's not despair I don't find the right word for it, only somehow that oh no how confused all this is, how has my life become like this, why can't everything be clear [...]

There is, however, a notable difference between Mari's and Susanna's responses to the therapists' invitation to consider what is going on in their minds. While Mari restricts herself to give an exposition of somehow alien forces ("you just shake," "you get scared") or external circumstances ("my body reacted really crazy to drinking coffee") having an impact on her, Susanna is talking about her "confusion," a state with more psychological meaning, albeit still somehow foreign and difficult to grasp.

Tanja, talking with Miina, a 39-year-old medical student who sought help for her painful emotional aftermaths of her divorce, showed a different discursive strategy of evoking in her client a self-exploring stance. She affiliated with Miina's emotional experience, and as a result the possibility of exploring Miina's own way of relating to her feelings was opened:

> Tanja: *they sound terrible painful those feelings you are living with*
>
> Miina: but then I wonder that when I have had also this thought that are they kind of real these feelings or am I only manipulating others by giving the impression that I am like this, that I have this bad feeling, is this only some fraud
>
> Tanja: *what do you mean by manipulation*
>
> [...]
>
> Miina: that is this only that I get attention when I
>
> Tanja: *that is this my own feeling*

Tanja's turns, first an affiliation ("the feelings sound terrible painful") showing a stance of empathy, second asking for clarification ("what do you mean by manipulation"), and third a formulation of the client's dilemma ("is this my own feeling") are all representative instances of the use of the therapeutic discourse. They serve to elicit a self-observing position for the client and open the possibility for further exploration of her way of constructing her emotional experience. Note that here there is no reference to "the mind" as the place where the emotions reside. Tarja did a similar work of exploring Laura's emotional experience by offering different labels of emotions:

Tarja: *was it, was it more of that kind of anger or disappointment*
Laura: well, when I was just that
Tarja: *or sorrow or*
Laura: by me you mean [*yes*] perhaps in a way disappointment and then I thought that now once again

Laura has told about her husband's untoward behavior and Tarja is asking about her emotional response. Tarja's way of proposing different possible emotional states constructs for her a position of somebody knowable of such potential states, a typical achievement of the use of the therapeutic discourse. Such a position is appropriate for somebody in the psychotherapist's role and does not in this context appear as arrogant or patronizing.

Talking About Goals and Tasks

Naturally, one central topic of these first meetings between clients and therapists was to formulate and negotiate a shared, even if tentative, understanding of the goal and tasks of the therapeutic work. This was contributed to by clients and therapists alike. There was a wide range of ways in which the goals of the treatment were expressed and formulated. The clients could give short metaphorical illustrations of what they wanted to achieve or they could formulate quite extensive agendas for the therapy. Some of the therapists, but not all, explicated their own understandings of what the therapeutic work would focus on and attempt to achieve.

Interestingly, getting rid of disturbing symptoms and alleviation of psychological distress were frequently offered as reasons of entering psychotherapy, but seldom expressed, either by clients or therapists, as actual goals of the therapeutic work. Rather, when formulating treatment goals, which could be done in quite colloquial ways or in rather elaborated wordings, the clients' central desire was usually to reach more understanding of their difficulties. Most of the therapists, in these first encounters, refrained from expressing their own views on the goals of the treatment, only in a couple of cases did the therapist give a clear statement of his/her position in this respect.

Adopting a colloquial discourse, some clients used metaphorical expressions when articulating their goals:

Helena: one should get all the pieces of the puzzle together
Miina: I thought that if one would try to fix one's noodle
Laura: they are just there in some lump all the issues ((I need to work on))

Such expressions, drawing upon a cultural stock of figurative speech, gave the encounter a flavor of mundanity and easiness, concealing possible tensions or apprehensions. Eija, again, formulated a quite articulated agenda for her treatment when responding to Tarja's invitation:

Tarja: *how could I help you*
Eija: well, I had such an idea that those issues have somehow to be spoken about that ((arise)) from childhood, surely connected to these fears and somehow disappointments in oneself [*yeah*] and then also the violent partner relation, what it has done to me [...] and how all this connects to this secrecy in life today and that kind of feeling of shame

Tarja's turn is typical for the kinds of opening lines used by the therapists early in the sessions. Eija's response, connecting personal history to present psychological difficulties, exhibits an advanced preunderstanding of what therapeutic work might entail, not wholly uncommon to the clients in this data. Later in the session, Tarja gave a formulation of the goal of the treatment typical for therapeutic discourse. The way she put it highlighted self-understanding, self-efficacy, and an autonomous attitude as universal goals of psychotherapy:

Tarja: *a good goal could be that you would get some kind of power and belief somehow in yourself, that you would to such an extend get to know yourself that you would dare to be yourself in those situations and, how would I say* [mm], *would start from your own needs and feelings, rather than that you adjust to what somebody else wants*

In a similar vein, Tero articulated for Mari his view on the goals for the psychotherapy. In his wording self-actualization and self-worth were raised as essential therapeutic goals:

> Tero: [...] *one could from that point of view say that therapy would be something by which you could become more yourself, become Mari, and stand like on your own ground trusting that you as a human person, as Mari, are valuable and* [...]

It should be noted, though, that such elaborate articulation of therapeutic goals, given by therapists, was not common in the data. Rather, most therapists contended themselves with subscribing to goals as formulated by the clients.

Constructing Reformulations of the Client's Problems

Considering that these were the first sessions of therapies, expected by clients and therapists alike to be rather long (the range of actualized sessions was from 19 to 57), it is not surprising that discursive exchanges explicitly targeted at therapeutic transformations were not frequent in the data. The conversations included only a few instances where therapeutic discourse was used to design actual therapeutic interventions, aiming at changing the client's understandings, attributions, or attitudes towards self or others. Speech with an intention to boost the clients' motivation for being involved in therapeutic efforts was also scarce.

In their session, Tero and Mari renegotiated—in colloquial discourse—the meaning of Mari's "sensitivity":

> Mari: I might have been starting to think that it ((the sensitivity)) could be a little bit a part of my nature that [*yeah*] I have somewhat been like that
>
> Tero: *yes, yes we are sensitive in different ways* [mm] *but that sensitivity of course wouldn't necessarily have to be such a negative thing*
>
> Mari: mm, yes like that I do want to be sensitive, that's why I actually didn't want to take the antidepressants, because I thought that from them you get that kind of feeling, and because I draw and paint it is not in that

way a bad thing, so in that way I'm even proud of it but still I wouldn't like to have these kinds of symptoms

In his response to Mari's turn, Tero questions her negative connotation of her sensitivity by, first, stating sensitivity to be a common characteristic of people and, second, by challenging softly ("of course," "not necessarily") the negative meaning of the word. Using a more deliberate therapeutic strategy, Tea pinpointed a positive exception in Anna's, a 21-year-old student, problematic habit to vomit after binging, which was referred to in colloquial terms as a "routine":

Tea: *it has become some kind of a routine*

Anna: yeah, and that is like the most terrible thing how morbid a routine one can have

Tea: *but when I heard you, it is however so that now eight days is quite a long time* [yes], *that you have anyway even that long managed to be without vomiting*

Tea disregards Anna's characterization of her habit as "morbid" and redirects the topicalization of the matter to Anna's achievement of having broken the habit for a period over many days. Tuula, in her session with Helena, offered a more radical reformulation of her client's problematic experience:

Helena: so you kind of adjusted yourself and were flexible and took all the chores that my sister left undone and so on [*yeah*], somehow you surely adapted to the role of a nice girl [*mm*] quite strongly

Tuula: *have you now, by falling ill with not carrying out things, revolted here now, that now I don't want to be like this*

Helena: something like this it could be

Tuula: *well, it just came here to my mind that*

Helena: or at least I would like to learn to defend myself and so

Tuula: *that people do things like that*

Using passive voice ("you"), Helena describes how she adopted a submissive role ("a nice girl") in her family. Tuula responds to this by suggesting, in the form of a question, that Helena's "illness" actually could be understood as a "revolt," and as such as something understandable, not uncommon, and perhaps even desirable. The reformulation is strengthened by paraphrasing Helena's potential inner dialogue—"I don't want to be like this." The uptake on Helena's side is positive and results in her formulating a personal goal for change.

Conclusions

To explore how psychotherapy could be approached as a specific mode of social practice, I analyzed, using a discursive perspective, the first sessions of nine individual psychotherapies, conducted by five different therapists. How did the clients and therapists fashion their conversational exchange? What were the topics? What forms of speech—types of discourses—were in use? What were the common features of the conversations in this respect? How did they differ from each other? What can be concluded—or at least suggested—about psychotherapy as social activity from this data and analysis?

Six topical themes that were dealt with by all the client-therapist dyads were found. These included talking about the client's problematic experience, the possible reasons for his/her problems, the relational context of the session, goals and tasks of the therapy, the psychology of the client's mind, and alternative ways to formulate and relate to the client's problems. Three different forms of speech—the medical, the colloquial, and the therapeutic discourse—were identified. The colloquial discourse, the use of mundane words and expressions, was the one used most by the interlocutors. The medical discourse, the use of professional terminologies from psychiatry and clinical psychology, was the one used the least and only when dealing with the presenting problem. The therapeutic discourse was used mostly by therapists but also by some of the clients, and introduced vocabularies and expressions by which the clients' experiences, attitudes, and other mind-related phenomena could be discussed, as well as issues related to the therapy as a form of treatment.

It seems fair to conclude that the client-therapist dyads did not seek to establish the sessions as any kind of expert consultation on the client's problems. The therapists did not primarily inquire about facts; they were rather interested in the subjective meanings the clients gave to their difficulties. When the clients gave detailed factual descriptions of their problems, these appeared to function primarily as evidence for the suffering of the client, not as markers indicating the nature of the problem. The presenting problem was not, by either counterpart, treated mainly as an indicator of some specific mental health disorder but sooner as an experience carrying personal meanings and a problem connected to the world of their everyday lives (Dreier, 2015).

Although colloquial language was the preferred speech genre used by the interlocutors, this did not mean that the conversations would not have features that would make them stand out as a particular form of social practice. These features correspond to some earlier findings from discursive and conversational research on psychotherapeutic encounters. Using mixtures of therapeutic and colloquial discourse, the therapeutic dyads constructed a shared observational position (Leiman, 2012) from where to look at the psychology of the client's mind. This discursive achievement also indicated the possibility and entitlement of the therapist to have access to some operations of the client's mind, not accessible to the client him- or herself (Weiste, Voutilainen, & Peräkylä, 2015).

An interesting observation was that an elaborated use of therapeutic discourse seemed to be counterproductive to the construction of a shared observer's position. This is in line with the notion of a therapeutic zone of proximal development (Leiman & Stiles, 2001), within which the therapist should move, not to lose contact to the client's linguistic domain. The use of colloquial vocabulary and shared metaphorical expressions could be seen to be instrumental in this respect. Likewise, as shown earlier by Penttinen, Wahlström, and Hartikainen (2016), displaying empathy and affiliation with the client's emotional experience served to help the client to take a reflective stance towards his/her way of relating to the problematic experience.

In summary then, one can conclude that the findings from the present analysis support Wampold's and Imel's (2015) notion of a contextual meta-model for understanding how psychotherapy works. Of the three pathways to therapeutic effect, suggested by that model, the first one, founding a real personal relationship, was clearly visible in the data. The frequent use of colloquial discourse emphasized the establishment of a person-to-person relationship between client and therapist as a primary function of these encounters. When therapists and clients shared the use of common expressions within the frame of a professional encounter, they appeared to create a quite distinct social context where intimate experiences could be approached from novel perspectives. This may be the discursive basis for what Gelso (2009) calls "the real relationship"—in his system one of three elements of the therapeutic relationship (the two others being the therapeutic alliance and the transference-countertransference configurations). In view of the dominance of the colloquial discourse in this data, the function of this speech genre in therapeutic encounters is clearly worth more research.

Considering the second pathway, creating an expectation of beneficial effect, the therapists in this data appeared to be cautious of not giving the clients a too optimistic view of the benefits of the treatment, as if thus seeking to ensure the clients' true engagement in the future efforts. Not surprisingly, the third pathway, concrete therapeutic actions, was still not frequent in these first sessions. The main actual therapeutic action in which the dyads engrossed in was the budding construction of a shared observational and reflective stance towards the client's problematic experience and his/her way of relating to it. What this study shows is that each of the pathways of the contextual model is realized in a large variety of discursive acts and deserves a detailed exploration. Building the relationship, creating hope, and engaging the client in useful new ways of action can be achieved in many ways but always include the mutual efforts of therapists and clients.

This analysis of therapy-talk aimed primarily to be descriptive. Undoubtedly some of the discursive practices applied by the therapists were more productive than others from the perspective of therapeutic progress. It is, however, outside the scope of this chapter to make a systematic appraisal of the therapists' talk turns in this respect. What the chapter does contribute—hopefully—is an approach to looking at the actual events of therapy conversations and the importance of discursive usages and details which are significant, and often even consequential for the practice, but frequently overlooked in clinical textbooks and guidelines. The transferability of the observations to other cultural contexts may be limited, but the approach itself can afford clinical practitioners and researchers alike an encouragement to take a fresh look at how therapists and clients together make psychotherapy happen.

References

Avdi, E., & Georgaca, E. (2007). Discourse analysis and psychotherapy: A critical review. *European Journal of Psychotherapy and Counselling, 9*, 157–176. https://doi.org/10.1080/13642530701363445

Dreier, O. (2015). Interventions in everyday lives: How clients use psychotherapy outside their sessions. *European Journal of Psychotherapy & Counselling, 17*, 114–128. https://doi.org/10.1080/13642537.2015.1027781

Gelso, C. J. (2009). The real relationship in a postmodern world: Theoretical and empirical explorations. *Psychotherapy Research, 19*, 253–264. https://doi.org/10.1080/10503300802389242

Harper, D. (2006). Discourse analysis. In M. Slade & S. Priebe (Eds.), *Choosing methods in mental health research: Mental health research from theory to practice* (pp. 47–67). London, UK: Routledge.

Leiman, M. (2012). Dialogical sequence analysis in studying psychotherapeutic discourse. *International Journal for Dialogical Science, 6*, 123–147.

Leiman, M., & Stiles, W. B. (2001). Dialogical sequence analysis and the zone of proximal development as conceptual enhancements to the assimilation model: The case of Jan revisited. *Psychotherapy Research, 11*, 311–330. https://doi.org/10.1080/713663986

Mayring, P. (2014). *Qualitative content analysis: Theoretical foundation, basic procedures and software solution.* Retrieved from http://www.psychopen.eu/fileadmin/user_upload/books/mayring/ssoar-2014-mayring-Qualitative_content_analysis_theoretical_foundation.pdf

Penttinen, H., Wahlström, J., & Hartikainen, K. (2016). Assimilation, reflexivity, and therapist responsiveness in group psychotherapy for social phobia: A case study. *Psychotherapy Research, 27*, 710–772. https://doi.org/10.1080/10503307.2016.1158430

Potter, J. (2003). Discourse analysis and discursive psychology. In P. M. Camic, J. E. Rhodes, & L. Yardley (Eds.), *Qualitative research in psychology: Expanding perspectives in methodology and design* (pp. 73–94). Washington, DC: American Psychological Association.

Taylor, C. (2016). *The language animal: The full shape of the human linguistic capacity*. Cambridge, MA: Harvard University Press.

Wahlström, J. (2006). The narrative metaphor and the quest for integration in psychotherapy. In E. O'Leary & M. Murphy (Eds.), *New approaches to integration in psychotherapy* (pp. 38–49). London, UK: Routledge.

Wampold, B. E. (2001). *The great psychotherapy debate. Models, methods and findings*. Mahwah, NJ: Lawrence Erlbaum Associates.

Wampold, B. E., & Imel, Z. E. (2015). *The great psychotherapy debate: The evidence for what makes psychotherapy work*. New York, NY: Routledge.

Weiste, E., Voutilainen, L., & Peräkylä, A. (2015). Epistemic asymmetries in psychotherapy interaction: Therapists' practices for displaying access to clients' inner experiences. *Sociology of Health and Illness, 38*, 645–661. https://doi.org/10.1111/1467-9566.12384

Wiggins, S. (2017). *Discursive psychology: Theory, method and applications*. London, UK: Sage.

3

Researching the Discursive Construction of Subjectivity in Psychotherapy

Evrinomy Avdi and Eugenie Georgaca

In this chapter, we explore the potential of discursive research for studying the interactional processes through which subjectivity is constituted, negotiated, and reformulated within and through the psychotherapeutic dialogue. We argue for the usefulness of the concept of subject positioning as a means for studying how subjectivity is talked into being in therapeutic conversations, while recognizing that psychotherapeutic conversations can provide rich material for social constructionist analyses of contemporary ideologies regarding selfhood and their intersections

We would like to dedicate this chapter to the memory of Michael Guilfoyle, esteemed colleague and friend, whose work continues to inspire us.

E. Avdi (✉) • E. Georgaca
School of Psychology, Aristotle University of Thessaloniki, Thessaloniki, Greece
e-mail: avdie@psy.auth.gr; georgaca@psy.auth.gr

O. Smoliak, T. Strong (eds.), *Therapy as Discourse*, The Language of Mental Health,
https://doi.org/10.1007/978-3-319-93067-1_3

with discourses around gender, family values, parenthood, mental health, and so on.

Initially, we present our perspective on psychotherapy as discursive practice, outline the main ways in which subjectivity has been conceptualized in social constructionist accounts, introduce the concept of subject positioning, and provide a selective review of discursive research on psychotherapy with a focus on the study of subjectivity. Next, we illustrate the potential of discursive research for understanding how subjectivity is transformed within therapy through an example of analysis of part of a session from a couple therapy. Finally, we discuss the theoretical, clinical, and research implications of this body of work.

Social Constructionism and Psychotherapy

In line with constructionist principles, we approach psychotherapy as a discourse and a set of practices, which rely upon the so-called psy-complex, the set of professional concepts and practices that promote a psychological understanding of human life (Pulido-Martinez, 2014), that has become increasingly pertinent, over the course of the twentieth century, in constructing personhood and in regulating social and emotional life in Western cultures (e.g. Parker, 1994). Within this framework, psychotherapy is conceptualized as a primarily semantic process, that is, a process of meaning construction, that simultaneously relies upon and promotes psychological understandings of life and human subjectivity. The intersections and cross-fertilizations between social constructionism and psychotherapy have a relatively long history; starting from the articulation of psychotherapy approaches explicitly committed to the turn to language and post-structuralism, the concepts of narrative, dialogue, and discourse have become key metaphors in the majority of traditional psychotherapy schools, while the focus on meaning co-construction is increasingly recognized as a potential unifying paradigm in psychotherapy (e.g. Wahlström, 2006). Although not a unitary field, discursively informed approaches to psychotherapy share an assumption that psychological distress is associated with limited and limiting self-narratives, in the sense that aspects of lived experience remain poorly discursively articulated or articulated in ways that maintain problem-saturated subject positions. Furthermore, it is assumed that problem-saturated constructions often have an ideological dimension, in the sense that they are shaped by, and accordingly sustain, culturally preferred discourses. Correspondingly, discursively informed psychotherapy aims to expand or reconstruct problem-focused constructions of the client's life and subjectivity and facilitate the discursive articulation of inclusive, polyphonic, and empowering self-narratives.

Despite recent developments in discursive theory and practice, discursive research occupies a relatively small place—in both numbers and scope—within the psychotherapy research literature. This could be attributed to several different factors, including theoretical/epistemological (the positivist bias of psychotherapy research), political/economical (selective funding for outcome studies, aligned with the "drug metaphor") theoretical/methodological (challenges of post-structuralist research), as well as the fact that many social constructionist researchers assume a critical position towards psychotherapy as an institution.

In our earlier work, we reviewed discursive studies on psychotherapy and suggested that discursive research can contribute to our understanding of how the meaning of the problem and clients' subjectivity are negotiated and transformed within psychotherapy talk; we also argued that discursive research provides rich, detailed, and critical analyses of the process of psychotherapy, thus potentially promoting clinically relevant research (Avdi & Georgaca, 2007, 2009). Since that time, discursive research on psychotherapy has grown, as a small but increasing number of researchers utilize discourse and conversation analysis to study their own and others' practice. In this chapter, we do not aim to review this literature comprehensively, but selectively discuss work that focuses on the manifestation and reformulation of subjectivity in therapy talk.

Social Constructionist Accounts of Personhood and the Concept of Subjectivity

Mainstream psychological accounts of selfhood tend to represent the self as an identifiable, stable, internally consistent, and self-contained entity. These psychological accounts reflect the ideal of "self-contained individualism," which arguably constitutes the dominant version of personhood in contemporary Western cultures (Sampson, 2003), and which approaches the "self" as an independent, undivided, unitary subject, a center of motivation and agency that is clearly demarcated from its social context. Over the last decades, these conceptualizations have been powerfully critiqued from several different perspectives, as naïve realist, essentialist, individualizing, culturally specific, and ethically problematic (e.g. Henriques, Hollway, Urwin, Venn, & Walkerdine, 1998). In this chapter, we use the term "subjectivity" to denote subjective experience and one's sense of self, and we assume that this is constituted in and through language and social interaction. From this perspective, subjectivity is situated, contextualized, variable, and shaped by ideology and power dynamics, yet also affectively charged, private, and intimately personal.

Currently, there is not one, unified discursive theory of subjectivity, as discursive accounts draw upon different traditions, including Althusser's interpellation theory, psychoanalysis, post-structuralism, and feminism (e.g. Törrönen, 2001), and this theoretical multiplicity is reflected in the different ways in which subjectivity is conceptualized and studied in discursive studies of psychotherapy. In terms of theory, a shared element of discursive approaches is the focus on language as constructive, functional, and variable; as such, discursive studies tend to examine the processes through which reality, agency, and accountability are created and negotiated within interaction. Consequently, subjectivity in discursive accounts is approached as jointly constructed in situated interactions and shaped by culturally available systems of meaning (e.g. Avdi & Georgaca, 2009).

A key concept for examining subjectivity in discursive approaches is subject positioning (Davies & Harré, 1990; Harré & van Langenhove, 1998). Subject positioning can be broadly described in terms of two interrelated, yet distinct, levels. On the one hand, it underscores the relational and interactional nature of subjectivity and refers to the position one assumes in specific interactions. When we speak, we assume a specific position and each story we tell is also—more or less explicitly—a story about who we are. We tell a different story of our troubles, for example, when we assume the position of a concerned parent, a troubled adolescent, or a mentally ill patient. Furthermore, each utterance is always addressed to someone, who we thus "call into" a particular position; the other can in turn accept, resist, challenge, or change this position invitation, and through his or her response, he or she in turn positions us (Drewery, 2005) in an ongoing process that constitutes the dynamics of the interaction. These exchanges are context-dependent and imbued with power, in the sense that in some contexts some participants have more say in positioning others, while some positions may be harder to resist. In psychotherapy, for example, the institutional position of "therapist" has more say in both defining meaning and in regulating the sequence of interaction than that of "client." From this perspective, our habitual positionings—which can be distressing, painful, or problem-saturated—are maintained through our interactions with a "community of subjection" (Guilfoyle, 2014), that is, significant others in our life who, often unwittingly, participate in our interpellation in problematic subject positions, enforcing norms associated with dominant discourses. Furthermore, when taking one position, we automatically do not take another; this selective positioning is relevant to psychotherapy, as clients can be seen to repetitively assuming problematic subject positions, while disavowing aspects of their potential multiplicity.

In terms of analysis, we can examine positioning in therapy whenever a participant speaks, is addressed to or is spoken about, through questions such as: Who speaks? In whose name do they speak? Who do they address? Who do they speak for? Different positions entail differing degrees of accountability and can have a variety of functions in the interaction, such as attributing blame or refuting an unwanted identity (Georgaca & Avdi, 2011). In sum, from a perspective that focuses on the performative and functional aspects of language use, positioning is a key process through which selves are performed, jointly constructed—and potentially reconstructed—through language and within interaction. Psychotherapy, in this framework, works through creating a particular type of conversation within which the problematic or distressing subject positions clients occupy are explored, challenged, or expanded.

The second level of conceptualizing subject positioning focuses on the intersection between ideology, power/knowledge, and subjectivity; this level concerns the location of the person in discourse and within a moral order (Harré & van Langenhove, 1998) and the focus is on the ways in which speakers are positioned through particular discourses. This perspective draws primarily upon Foucault's work and assumes that discourses entail an array of subject positions that people take up when they talk; these positions influence the course of interactions, the actions available to people, as well as their sense of self (Parker, 1994). Furthermore, these processes often take place irrespective of speakers' intentions and outside of awareness. For example, when a psychotherapist meets a client, the way each participant interacts and experiences him- or herself is influenced not only by their individual biographies, but is also powerfully shaped by their respective, institutionally sanctioned positions of "therapist" and "client," each of which has specific claims to knowledge and authority. As mentioned above, subject positions are closely implicated with power/knowledge; power here is approached as a constitutive force, closely associated with specific sets of knowledge that maintain their status through disqualifying alternative knowledge and naturalizing dominant discourses. As such, when deploying a particular discourse and its associated subject positions, we are implicated in an—often implicit—power struggle over the meanings that are seen as normal, good, and true. In terms of analysis, subject positioning on this level can be explored through investigating the discourses that are implicated in clients' and therapists' talk and identifying the subject positions thus rendered available.

In sum, discursive accounts propose that identity has no stable essence but is constituted within interactions and consists of a multiplicity of—more or less transiently held—subject positions. Different subject positions are associated with rhetorical devices that place oneself and the other in different relations, for example, relations of power, competence, knowledge, moral standing, and so on, and these positions are created within the context of existing, culturally provided categories and storylines (Harré & van Langenhove, 1998).

Discursive accounts underscore the multiplicity, fluidity, and fragmentation of subjectivity, in contrast to most psychological accounts that focus on the integrity and coherence of self-identity. This tendency has been criticized for losing touch with the phenomenological and experiential realities of everyday living, whereby most of us experience our self as having a sense of continuity in time and across situations. Lived experience would suggest that subjects may be discursively decentered, that is, multiply positioned, as suggested by positioning theory, but phenomenologically centered, that is, experienced as defined by internal processes and with a limited range of positions available (Guilfoyle, 2014). Indeed, discursive theorizing cannot readily account for the observation that people tend to inhabit specific subject positions, often holding on to them rigidly and with great tenacity, such that any shift in positioning seems difficult to achieve. To address this observation, several authors combined psychoanalysis with discursive analyses to explain individuals' unconscious investment in specific subject positions (e.g. Frosh, Phoenix, & Pattman, 2003; Georgaca, 2005; Hollway & Jefferson, 2000), while others examined identifications with specific subject positions in terms of ideology and power drawing upon Foucault and post-Foucauldian theories (e.g. Guilfoyle, 2014). Despite these attempts, the dynamics and processes through which individuals tend to repetitively deploy an—often limited—range of subject positions are not fully addressed within discursive theorizing.

Related to the above, another contentious issue in discursive theories of subjectivity concerns so-called discourse determinism, that is, the assumption that culturally available discourses define experience and identity. This has been criticized for producing a version of "blank subjectivity" (Parker, 1994) and failing to account for changes in positioning, agency, and resistance to the power of discourse. Several authors agree that subjects are constituted by discourse but not completely subjected to its power; this brings forth questions regarding the nature of that which lies outside discourse and resists its power that have not been fully addressed in constructionist theory.

Finally, the almost exclusive focus on language has been criticized for sidestepping the embodied aspects of human life as well as the role of the material environment in the processes of social construction; we discuss embodied aspects of positioning in more depth in the next section.

Extra-discursive Aspects of Positioning

In recent years, several authors have increasingly commented on the limits of positioning theory in describing the embodied and affective aspect of human life and argue that our sense of self, the experience of distress, and the processes implicated in social construction are always embodied (e.g. Cromby, 2012). In these accounts, subject positioning is considered a corporeal as well as a discursive accomplishment, as the subject is seen to be constituted through joint actions that take place in situated, embodied, and material contexts (e.g. Shotter, 1993). In this framework, embodied and affective processes are not conceptualized as independent of culture and discourse but as distinct, dynamic processes that are inscribed in discourse (e.g. Burkitt, 2014; Wetherell, 2015).

Research on communication suggests that face-to-face dialogue takes place through the intertwined cooperation of different modalities (speech, facial expression, gesture, gaze, body posture, prosody, and aspects of the material surroundings) that work together to create meaning (e.g. Goodwin, 2000). Discursive analyses can discern some aspects of non-verbal positioning through examining the form and organization of talk (e.g. shifts in footing, pauses, hesitations, etc.) but some aspects of the construction of subjectivity arguably take place outside the verbal realm; this is a point not yet adequately addressed in discursive research. Moreover, expanding our conceptualization of positioning to include extra-discursive aspects creates tensions on both theoretical and methodological levels that have only recently begun to be systematically addressed in the constructionist literature (e.g. Wetherell, 2015). Below, we briefly outline some literature that we consider could help expand our conceptualizations of subject positioning to include non-verbal and embodied aspects.

Although recognized as important, prosodic and other non-verbal aspects of talk are rarely analyzed systematically in discursive studies, with a few exceptions (e.g. Tomicic, Martinez, & Krause, 2014; Weiste & Peräkylä, 2014). These studies have shown that prosody plays an important role in creating meaning and in mutual positioning, independently from the content of talk. Even more difficult to incorporate in discursive analyses are visuo-spatial aspects of communication, for example, gesture, facial expression, orientation, and so on. Starting with Freud's view of symptoms as symbolic expression of underlying unconscious conflict, several theories contend that un-narrated experiences are "told" through the body or through action.

Recent knowledge about procedural memory and implicit relational knowledge has provided a basis for the assumption that some aspects of experience may be potentially unsayable (e.g. Cromby & Harper, 2009). A few discursive studies have started to include non-verbal aspects of communication in their analyses (e.g. Bavelas, McGee, Phillips, & Routledge, 2000) but none have done so in a systematic manner in the context of psychotherapy. Moreover, very few studies have attempted to examine silences or that which is not said in therapy (e.g. Itävuori et al., 2015).

Another interesting development includes the study of the embodied aspects of co-construction as reflected in psychophysiological reactions. There is some evidence that processes of self-construction, identity negotiation, and positioning are associated with increases in autonomic arousal (e.g. Lyons & Cromby, 2010). Similarly, some recent studies found evidence for psychophysiological synchrony in interacting dyads during narration of emotionally laden stories (Peräkylä et al., 2015; Voutiläinen et al., 2014). Furthermore, few recent studies have attempted to link embodied aspects of interaction with meaning construction and positioning in psychotherapy, but this literature is still in its infancy (e.g. Päivinen et al., 2016; Seikkula, Karvonen, Kykyri, Kaartinen, & Penttonen, 2015).

In summarizing the above, social constructionism has provided a powerful critique of traditional accounts of the self but not a complete theory of personhood. Within this literature, there is an ongoing tension between the recognition of the interactional, situation-specific constitution of subjectivity, on the one hand, and the phenomenological experiences of continuity, coherence, and agency on the other. Also, despite the evidence that extra-discursive factors play an important role in human interactions, constructionist researchers and theoreticians have been rather slow in including the affective and embodied dimensions of human life in their study of interaction in therapy. At the same time, however, constructionist accounts have provided a powerful analytic tool, that of subject positioning, that can help us explore the relational and semantic processes through which identity is talked into being within psychotherapeutic conversations. In the next section, we selectively present and discuss studies that have used these tools to examine the reformulation of subjectivity in therapy.[1]

Discursive Research on Subjectivity in Psychotherapy

As already mentioned, discursive accounts approach subjectivity as multiple, variable, and fragmented; a key conceptualization of psychological difficulties arising from this perspective assumes that these are associated with a narrowing of the repertoire of available subject positions for the client, which constrains lived experience and limits options for action. Accordingly, therapy aims to enhance the clients' ability to flexibly adopt a wider range of subject positions. Following on from this, several discourse analyses examine the range of subject positions that clients employ in the course of therapy (e.g. Avdi, 2005; Frosh, Burck, Strickland-Clark, & Morgan, 1996), and it has been proposed that the *flexibility* with which clients position themselves in the therapy room can be used as a micro-outcome variable (Strong, Busch, & Couture, 2008) in psychotherapy research. Another aspect of the repertoire of available subject positions concerns the relationships between positions. For example, some of our subject positions are central to the way we define, experience, and present our self, and these tend to be in line with dominant ideologies. This dominance of some positions means that other subject positions may be thinly narrated, under-elaborated, or unassimilated. Indeed, some studies have shown that traumatic experiences, in particular, may remain unstoried and the corresponding subject positions unavailable, marginalized, or even dissociated (e.g. Bromberg, 1998). In such cases, the aim of therapy is that of fostering marginalized subject

[1] Over the last 15 years, there has been a flourishing of studies that utilize conversation analysis (CA) to study the process of psychotherapy (e.g. Peräkylä, Antaki, Vehviläinen, & Leudar, 2008; Sutherland & Strong, 2011); although we consider this body of work highly relevant to both psychotherapy research and clinical practice, we have not included it in this discussion, given that CA makes no reference to or claims about the speakers' internal processes or sense of self. Furthermore, we do not discuss studies that rely upon a dialogical perspective, as the majority of these hold a constructivist perspective and tend to focus on the client's talk studying subjectivity as an internal entity.

positions, thus expanding the person's position repertoire. To date, there are only a few discursive studies that explore the organization of the client's position repertoire, by examining, for example, the dynamics of dissociation and the degree of accessibility of different subject positions (e.g. Avdi, 2016; Guilfoyle, 2016). Finally, a few discursive studies have focused on the emergence through therapy of a superordinate, reflexive meta-position, that observes and talks about other subject positions (e.g. Georgaca, 2003).

A central issue in discursive research on therapy relates to *agency*. Several discursive studies have shown how clients manifest compromised agency, often associated with problem-saturated discourses, and have argued that therapeutic change is associated with clients coming to occupy more agentic positions; on the other hand, it has been argued that sometimes clients take on too much agency in the form of critical self-blame (Wahlström, 2006). Agency, however, is a thorny issue in social constructionist accounts; it has been problematized as reflecting the modernist psychological subject, and thus promoting an ahistorical, decontextualized, and over-psychologized representation of subjectivity (e.g. Henriques et al., 1998). On the other hand, agency is recognized as an important aspect of resistance to the dominance of discourse and, in many cases, an implicit aim of therapy.

Reflecting these theoretical tensions, the discursive studies that examine the negotiation of agency in therapy approach it in diverse ways. Some assume that agentic subject positions are indeed associated with psychological well-being and treat the emergence of increasingly agentic positions in the client's talk as evidence of therapeutic change (e.g. Burck, Frosh, Strickland-Clark, & Morgan, 1998). Others examine the interactional processes through which clients display weak agency, the rhetorical work through which agency is promoted, and the processes through which clients adopt more agentic positions, without discussing the ideological or practical implications of these practices (e.g. Madill & Doherty, 1994). Another group approach the construction of agentic subjects critically, as part of the ideology that promotes certain ideals regarding personhood, and illuminate the active role of therapists in producing "psychological subjects" in need of expert intervention (e.g. Guilfoyle, 2001).

The negotiation of agency has also been explored in relation to *accountability and responsibility for one's actions*. This is an issue that is particularly relevant in couple and family therapy, where questions around who the client is and who needs to change are often contentious and associated with blame (e.g. Avdi, 2015a; Kurri & Wahlström, 2005; Stancombe & White, 2005) as well as in situations where the client's actions are associated with morally delicate issues (e.g. Pärtanen, Wahlström, & Holma, 2006) or where the context of therapy is semi-mandatory (e.g. Seilonen, Wahlström, & Aaltonen, 2012).

Discursive research reveals the therapist's active role in promoting certain versions of reality and subjectivity, and this allows us to consider the ways in which specific sessions are embedded in wider systems of meaning, moral values, and ideology. Several discursive studies focus on *the role of dominant discourses* in the construction of particular versions of personhood. For example, several studies examine the implications of the medical discourse for the clients' agency; psychiatric conceptualizations have been shown to compound the person's experienced difficulties, as they provide pathological subject positions for the "patient" that constrain his or her agency, limit possibilities for action, and contribute to the person's alienation (e.g. Avdi, Lerou, & Seikkula, 2015; Karatza & Avdi, 2010). Children are another category of person that has been shown to be awarded half-membership status in therapy talk; for example, a series of studies have shown how children are simultaneously involved in and marginalized within family therapy practice (e.g. O'Reilly, 2008). These practices can be shown to be in line with discourses around child development and the claims to knowledge, rights, and responsibilities attributed to the categories of "child" and "adult" within these discourses (e.g. Avdi, 2015b). Other studies have focused on the effects on subjectivity of discourses around gender, explicating how these discourses create sexually divided subject positions (e.g. man/woman, father/mother, stepfather/stepmother, son/daughter, husband/wife) with specific rights and responsibilities, expected behaviors, as well as moral status and how these positions are intricately implicated with constructions of problems and their solutions (e.g. Suoninen & Wahlström, 2009).

In sum, in discursive studies, the difficulties that clients experience are often seen to arise from the use of a limited range of culturally dominant but pathologizing discourses, which restrict the range of subject positions that can be adopted. Accordingly, therapy is seen as a process of shifting the dominance of these discourses and enabling clients to adopt more varied subject positions, thus enriching the client's lived experience and sense of self. From this perspective, the role of a discursively aware therapist can be described as entailing, on the one hand, the deconstruction of dominant discourses that are implicated in problem-saturated subject positions for the client, and on the other hand, the co-construction of alternative discourses that sustain more empowering subject positions. This presupposes therapist flexibility in terms of discursive positioning and the conversational moves employed in the course of therapy, as well as the therapist assuming a meta-position of reflexive awareness of the complex, and power-imbued, discursive processes that take place in therapy.

Following this brief introduction to relevant theory and research, in the next section we present a brief analysis of an extract from one session of couple therapy, with an aim to illustrate the usefulness of a discursive approach to analysing the processes through which meanings and identities are negotiated in psychotherapy talk.

Case Analysis: Reformulating Meanings and Identities in Psychotherapy

The example we present is from a couple therapy that was conducted in a public mental health clinic in Greece, and the material was collected in the context of a broader research project.[2] All sessions were videotaped and permission has been granted for the use of the session material for research purposes. The therapy lasted 15 months, spanning over 15 sessions. There were two experienced female family therapists whose work included the use of a one-way mirror as well as reflecting conversations. The clients were a heterosexual, married couple. Both partners (Costas and Demetra) were white, Greek, in their mid-30s, and had been living

[2] Relational Mind in Events of Change in Multi-actor Therapeutic Dialogues—for an overview, see Seikkula et al. (2015).

together for several years before the birth of their son 10 months earlier. They came to couple therapy to resolve difficulties in their relationship that had intensified through conflicts in the division of labor following their transition to parenthood.

In this brief example of analysis, we focus on one of the issues in this therapy that concerns the difficulties Demetra experienced in the transition to motherhood; this was a highly emotive issue that dominated the initial sessions and was discussed throughout the therapy. We selectively focus on this topic, using material from the third session, to illustrate how the problem, initially diffuse and vaguely described, is gradually reformulated into a psychological issue that can be addressed in therapy—and note the therapist's active role in this process; we also illustrate how culturally preferred ideals are implicated in personal distress.

In the first session, Demetra reported struggling with the demands of caring for a young baby. She became very frustrated with the baby's demands, to such an extent that she often found herself screaming, kicking, and hurtling objects in rage. These outbursts were followed by intense guilt and her sense of being trapped in a terrible situation she could not manage. Early in the first session, she evocatively described how she sometimes felt like killing her baby, because his relentless demands for care led her to exhaustion.

Before turning to the extract, it is worth noting that Demetra's account is in stark contrast to culturally desirable and socially acceptable behaviors expected of mothers. Despite the powerful critique of dominant representations of motherhood articulated by feminist scholars for more than 30 years and the increasing recognition that motherhood is a multifaceted experience, ideals about motherhood abound and continue to influence women's experiences and identities, saturating everyday practices and interactions, and promoting social processes of gendered stratification (e.g. Goodwin & Huppatz, 2010). Images of "the good mother"—in the media, popular culture, public policy, and social institutions such as education and work—remain prevalent and continue to regulate women's lives, functioning as standards against which women are judged and judge themselves, as mothering continues to occupy a powerful position in women's identity (Arrendell, 2000). Contemporary feminist theorists have illuminated the diversity and flux that characterizes current representations of motherhood and have illustrated how such variations on a theme (e.g. the good working mother, the good lesbian mother, shared parenting, etc.) operate in different contexts with complex and sometimes contradictory effects, as they intersect with social processes related to social class, race, ethnicity, heteronormativity, as well as gender (Goodwin & Huppatz, 2010; Sévon, 2011).

In the analysis that follows, we focus on one aspect of the good motherhood ideology that is particularly relevant to this case. Feminist research has illuminated the prevalence of a discourse of *intensive mothering* in Western societies, which rests on the claim that mothering is exclusive, wholly child-centered, emotionally involving, and time-consuming (Hays, 1996). The subject position of good mother in this discourse is that of a self-sacrificing woman, devoted to the care of others, with no needs or desires of her own, an intuitive nurturer, naturally equipped and always readily available to care for her children, setting their needs as her exclusive priority. The intensive mothering ideology both assumes and reinforces traditional gender-based division of labor and an idealization of the nuclear family (Goodwin & Huppatz, 2010).

The interaction presented below took place in the middle of the third session, in which the focus was on Demetra's low mood and her sense entrapment. Until that point in the session, Demetra was reluctant to talk and responded to the therapist's attempts to engage her with single-word answers or with a simple "I don't know." She stated that her main problem related to feeling bored and finding little enjoyment in her life; she complained of having no time to herself, no social activities and few interests, and no sense that any change was possible. This diffuse, rather vague sense of distress and boredom dominated the discussion in the first half of the session. In terms of positioning, Demetra seems to simultaneously resist and adopt dominant discourses of mothering, which associate motherhood with personal fulfillment and happiness. The therapist's discursive agenda, that is, the overarching effects of her talk on the evolving conversation, can be seen to be that of reformulating this rather vague—and morally delicate—problem as a psychologically meaningful difficulty, while inviting Demetra in a less problematic and more agentic subject position. This is reflected in the therapist's persistence in exploring the possible meanings and causes of Demetra's experiences and providing links between her difficulties, her personal history, and dominant constructions of motherhood, evidenced in the extract below.

1	Th	*It seems like, especially you Demetra, like you are saying that, OK, you are bored with the things you used to do, it seems like you don't really have a wish to do other things, but (.) you are also crying (.) and this confuses me, what exactly are you crying about? (.) is this crying disappointment?*
2	D	*(5) I don't know [crying] (7) I don't know*
3	T	*Costas, do you know why Demetra is crying now? (.) Do you have a fantasy about it?*
4	C	*I don't want to*
5	T	*You don't want what?*
6	C	*To have a fantasy*
7	T	*Why?*
8	C	*Ehm, it is more dangerous*
9	T	*Dangerous?*
10	C	*Yes, better to know [laughter] what it is about*
11	T	*Mmm, Do you want to know?*
12	C	*Mmm, yes. Wouldn't I want to? (9)*
13	D	*I don't know [crying]*
14	C	*Mmm, OK, I didn't mean that you must tell me, when I said that I want to know*
15	D	*I generally feel, sometimes, that I am suffocating in this situation that (.) I don't want any more [crying] he pisses me off (.) I don't have any patience*
16	Th	*The baby?*
17	D	*Yes*
18	Th	*He pisses you off?*
19	D	*Hugely [cries] sometimes (.) I feel like throttling him (.) that would teach him (.) I don't have any patience*
20	Th	*He tires you, hmm?*
21	D	*Yes, he tires me, I don't know, I find it difficult to make the transition from the world of adults to this other world*

[brief interchange about the difficulties all adults have relating to babies]

22 Th *We talked about it briefly last time and I think that this is important (.) perhaps this has to do with an internal conflict you have between an imaginary, ideal mum and the mum that you actually are (…) to what extent would you allow yourself to sometimes be annoyed with a little creature who constantly demands (.) and to not be available? How likely is it that you'd allow yourself to experience this without feeling guilty (D- hardly at all [crying]) you wouldn't allow it at all?*

23 D *No, because when I get annoyed, I get annoyed (.) and I start shouting and screaming and kicking things, so that I don't bash him of course, so this is a very intense situation, it's not like "listen now, I am annoyed so calm down before…"*

24 Th *Hmm, perhaps you reach (.) you reach your limits*

25 D *It's not like "talk him through it," it's like (.) "go away, get away from me". The dog runs away, the child runs away, everyone runs away, like (.) this is like (.) mental illness [cries]*

26 Th *Who do you consider an ideal mum, Demetra? How did you, how do you imagine a perfect mum?*

27 D *I don't know [cries] My mum was a super-mum*
[brief discussion about Demetra's mother]

28 Th *What is your fantasy of the ideal mum? Because you are perhaps chasing that ideal and that's why you reach your limits*

29 D *Yeah, in this tv ad for (margarine brand), the one in the ad for (margarine brand) (.) who is tall, blonde, in superb shape, always smiling, with the perfectly laid table and the perfect breakfast, on time, and with perfect nails*

30 Th *Yes, but you know that this life exists only in ads (.) or don't you know that?*

31 D *Yeah (.) OK (.) this life exists only in ads*

32 Th *What I mean is, if there is a constant struggle inside you, about "what kind of mum am I? Am I a good mum or not?" and you set yourself such high standards, I understand that you get disappointed, because you feel that you are not the mum you'd like to be, and then it seems that everything else becomes boring*

In turn 1, the therapist summarizes Demetra's perspective about the problem (boredom and lack of interest) and then invites further elaboration of her experience by addressing Demetra's non-verbal expression of sadness. Until that point in the session, Demetra had been crying silently from time to time, but only responded briefly and non-committedly to the therapist's questions about this. Demetra seemed to be in a position of someone who is fed up with her life, exhausted, and withdrawn—with no agency or desire. Her experience seems under-narrated and stagnant, with no history to her troubles, no progression, and no causes or meanings associated with them. This subject position is both articulated and enacted in the interaction, as Demetra is a reluctant, un-cooperative client until that point. In her turn, the therapist marks Demetra's silent crying as puzzling ("it confuses me") and then suggests a possible psychological explanation for it (disappointment), thus inviting Demetra to elaborate. Demetra maintains a helpless position of someone who is in distress but does not know why.

There follows a brief interchange, where the therapist uses circular questioning and invites Costas to assume a position of observer of Demetra's distress. Costas responds from the position of partner, who addresses Demetra with gentleness and concern; in this way, Demetra is positioned as the primary client at this point in the session by both Costas and the therapist.

Interestingly, Demetra responds from the position of distressed mother, rather than that of a distressed partner, and starts to talk about her sense of entrapment, suffocation, and anger. We hypothesize that Demetra's rage and aggression towards her baby are delicate issues, as her feelings and actions are in sharp contrast to socially expected maternal behaviors; in a sense, she assumes a position of "bad mother." The therapist responds gently to this disclosure and Demetra describes her desire to "throttle" her baby.

The therapist ignores this strong statement and responds with a reformulation, reframing Demetra's aggression as fatigue. Reformulations are powerful discursive tools that selectively focus on one aspect of what has been said by the previous speaker or put a particular spin on it, thus changing the previous utterance while seemingly accepting it. They are commonly used rhetorical strategies in therapy talk that cast clients' complaints into the language of therapy (e.g. Davis, 1986; Buttny, 2004), and function to promote the reconstruction of the problem in line with the therapeutic agenda. As such, reformulations have an ideological dimension, in the sense that they promote a particular version of reality and subjectivity in line with therapeutic assumptions. In this case, through the therapist's reformulation, Demetra is called into the position of an exhausted rather than an aggressive mum; Demetra accepts this position call, which she elaborates upon introducing the difficulties in relating to babies. This new construction is further elaborated in turn 22, where the therapist introduces the idea of "internal conflict," a key notion in psychological discourse. At the same time, Demetra's initial account is altered quite significantly: the intensity of Demetra's aggression is toned down (she "sometimes" gets "annoyed" rather than "pissed off"), there are distancing markers ("you" don't allow "yourself" to experience such feelings) and a psychological explanation is provided that moderates the rage and takes attention off it (the problem is not Demetra's rage per se, but the fact that she doesn't allow herself to experience it). In this formulation, there is a very demanding little creature and an exhausted mum, who naturally sometimes gets annoyed; in this way, Demetra is positioned again as a good mum, who struggles because she tries to be perfect.

Demetra initially seems to accept this formulation but soon returns to the position of "bad mum," as she describes her anger as too intense and concludes that her response is abnormal ("mental illness"). The therapist again ignores this powerful statement and shifts topic; this shift is in line with her discursive agenda of constructing a non-pathological narrative, which is gradually built up into a complete interpretation in turn 32, and this interpretation becomes central in the remaining session. In turns 26–32, the therapist builds a formulation that links Demetra's difficulties with her high expectations that she constructs as resulting from her personal history (having a super mum) as well as from culturally dominant ideals about motherhood (TV advertisements). The therapist challenges both these constructions in a playful and humorous tone, an indication that she is managing a delicate issue (Buttny, 2004).

So, through this sequence of talk, the problem is reconstructed from boredom, to frustration and aggression, to psychological conflict and Demetra is re-positioned from a bad to a good mum, who is struggling because she tries to be perfect. Thus, the problem becomes one of perfectionism in relation to "false" ideas about motherhood rather than maternal aggression. The ideology around "perfect mums" and Demetra's "perfectionism" becomes the topic of conversation—and deconstruction—in the remaining session. In terms of discourses of motherhood, the therapist both invokes and deconstructs a caricature of ideal motherhood, which is consistent with the discourse of intensive mothering. At the same time, she brings forth a more moderate normative, discourse of motherhood, calling Demetra to assume a position within it and thus enabling a more acceptable subject position for her as a mother. It is worth noting that much less discursive work is performed in this therapy on Costas' corresponding position as father, and we consider this to reflect the relative power of motherhood discourses in defining and regulating women's subjectivity.

Discussion

It is clear from the discussion above that subjectivity is at the center of the psychotherapeutic process. Addressing the client's concerns in therapy always implicates issues of identity—including responsibility, agency, accountability, and morality—and so the meanings of the "problem" that brought the client to therapy are intricately implicated with how speakers position themselves and important others. In other words, the semantic work of psychotherapy entails "joint work on identity projects" (Wahlström, 2006) that often take the form of a negotiation and reformulation of the clients' identity, arguably in ways that open new avenues for experience and action.

We have argued, and demonstrated through the extract analysis, that the concept of subject positioning is a valuable tool for investigating the processes of reconstructing subjectivity in psychotherapy, as it enables the examination of the role both of interactional processes and of sociocultural discourses in shaping the client's self. We hope to have also demonstrated the importance of investigating the role of the therapist in actively shaping the psychotherapeutic process and thus forming particular, culturally and therapeutically preferred, client subject positions. In line with recent trends of discursive work on psychotherapy, we think that the non-verbal, affective, and bodily aspects of human life should be incorporated in discursive analyses of psychotherapy. While broadly acknowledging the non-verbal aspects of subject positioning, we regrettably have not been able to provide an analysis of non-verbal aspects of the brief interchange analyzed here. We certainly hope the analysis of subjectivity in psychotherapy in the future develops along these lines.

Finally, we hope to have demonstrated the relevance of positioning theory for clinical practice. We contend that recognizing the centrality of positioning for subjectivity, the multiplicity of positionings—for both therapists and clients—as well as the interactional, constructed, and context-bound character of positioning can enrich therapeutic understanding (Parker, 1999). We would argue that a distinctive feature of discursively informed approaches to therapy is attentiveness to the role of ideology and culturally dominant discourses in client distress. Accordingly, discursively aware therapists strive to exercise reflexive awareness of the discursive processes that constitute the process of therapy and flexibility in positioning within clinical conversations, in the service of deconstructing problematic discourses and opening up space for alternative discourses that enable the emergence of more empowering subject positions for the client.

References

Arrendell, T. (2000). Conceiving and investigating motherhood: The decade's scholarship. *Journal of Marriage and the Family, 62*, 1192–1207.

Avdi, E. (2005). Negotiating a pathological identity in the clinical dialogue. *Psychology and Psychotherapy: Theory, Research and Practice, 78*, 493–511.

Avdi, E. (2015a). Fostering dialogue: Exploring the therapists' discursive contributions in a couple therapy. In M. Borcsa & P. Rober (Eds.), *Research perspectives in couple therapy: Discursive qualitative methods* (pp. 71–88). Heidelberg: Springer.

Avdi, E. (2015b). Discourses of development in the consulting room: Analysing family therapy with children. *Feminism and Psychology, 25*(3), 363–380.

Avdi, E. (2016). Positioning as embodied interaction: Commentary on Guilfoyle. *Journal of Constructivist Psychology, 29*(2), 141–148.

Avdi, E., & Georgaca, E. (2007). Discourse analysis and psychotherapy: A critical review. *European Journal of Psychotherapy and Counselling, 9*(2), 157–176.
Avdi, E., & Georgaca, E. (2009). Narrative and discursive approaches to the analysis of subjectivity in psychotherapy. *Social and Personality Psychology Compass, 3*(5), 654–670.
Avdi, E., Lerou, V., & Seikkula, J. (2015). Dialogical features, therapist responsiveness and agency in a therapy for psychosis. *Journal of Constructivist Psychology, 28*(4), 329–341.
Bavelas, J. B., McGee, D., Phillips, B., & Routledge, R. (2000). Microanalysis of communication in psychotherapy. *Human Systems: The Journal of Systemic Consultation and Management, 11*(1), 3–22.
Bromberg, P. M. (1998). *Standing in the spaces: Essays on clinical process, trauma and dissociation*. London, UK: The Analytic Press.
Burck, C., Frosh, S., Strickland-Clark, L., & Morgan, K. (1998). The process of enabling change: A study of therapist interventions in family therapy. *Journal of Family Therapy, 20*, 253–267.
Burkitt, I. (2014). *Emotions and social relations*. London, UK: Sage.
Buttny, R. (2004). *Talking problems: Studies on discursive construction*. Albany: State University of New York Press.
Cromby, J. (2012). Narrative, discourse, psychotherapy—Neuroscience? In A. Lock & T. Strong (Eds.), *Discursive perspectives in therapeutic practice* (pp. 288–317). Oxford, UK: Oxford University Press.
Cromby, J., & Harper, D. (2009). Paranoia: A social account. *Theory and Psychology, 19*(3), 335–361.
Davies, B., & Harré, R. (1990). Positioning: The discursive production of selves. *Journal for the Theory of Social Behaviour, 20*(1), 43–63.
Davis, K. (1986). The process of problem re(formulation) in psychotherapy. *Sociology of Health and Illness, 8*, 44–74.
Drewery, W. (2005). Why we should watch what we say: Position calls, everyday speech, and the production of relational subjectivity. *Theory & Psychology, 15*(3), 305–324.
Frosh, S., Burck, C., Strickland-Clark, L., & Morgan, K. (1996). Engaging with change: A process study of family therapy. *Journal of Family Therapy, 18*, 141–161.
Frosh, S., Phoenix, A., & Pattman, R. (2003). Taking a stand: Using psychoanalysis to explore the positioning of subjects in discourse. *British Journal of Social Psychology, 42*, 39–53.
Georgaca, E. (2003). Exploring signs and voices in the therapeutic space. *Theory & Psychology, 13*(4), 541–560.

Georgaca, E. (2005). Lacanian psychoanalysis and the subject of social constructionist psychology: Analysing subjectivity in talk. *International Journal of Critical Psychology, 14*, 74–94.

Georgaca, E., & Avdi, E. (2011). Discourse analysis. In D. J. Harper & A. Thompson (Eds.), *Qualitative research methods in mental health and psychotherapy: An introduction for students and practitioners* (pp. 147–162). Chichester, UK: Wiley.

Goodwin, C. (2000). Action and embodiment within situated human interaction. *Journal of Pragmatics, 32*, 1489–1522.

Goodwin, S., & Huppatz, K. (Eds.). (2010). *The good mother: Contemporary motherhoods in Australia*. Sydney: Sydney University Press.

Guilfoyle, M. (2001). Problematizing psychotherapy: The discursive production of a bulimic. *Culture and Psychology, 7*, 151–179.

Guilfoyle, M. (2014). *The person in narrative therapy: A post-structuralist Foucauldian account*. London, UK: Palgrave Macmillan.

Guilfoyle, M. (2016). Subject positioning: Gaps and stability in the therapeutic encounter. *Journal of Constructivist Psychology, 29*(2), 123–140.

Harré, R., & van Langenhove, L. (1998). *Positioning theory*. London, UK: Wiley Blackwell.

Hays, S. (1996). *The cultural contradictions of motherhood*. New Haven, CT: Yale University Press.

Henriques, J., Hollway, W., Urwin, C., Venn, C., & Walkerdine, V. (1998). *Changing the subject* (2nd ed.). London, UK: Routledge.

Hollway, W., & Jefferson, T. (2000). *Doing qualitative research differently*. London, UK: Sage.

Itävuori, S., Korvela, E., Karvonen, A., Penttonen, M., Kaartinen, J., Kykyri, V. L., et al. (2015). The significance of silent moments in creating words for the not-yet-spoken experiences in threat of divorce. *Psychology, 6*(11), 1360–1372.

Karatza, H., & Avdi, E. (2010). Shifts in subjectivity during the therapy for psychosis. *Psychology and Psychotherapy: Theory, Research and Practice, 84*(2), 214–229.

Kurri, K., & Wahlström, J. (2005). Placement of responsibility and moral reasoning in couple therapy. *Journal of Family Therapy, 27*, 352–369.

Lyons, A., & Cromby, J. (2010). Social psychology and the empirical body: Rethinking the relationship. *Social and Personality Psychology Compass, 4*(1), 1–13.

Madill, A., & Doherty, K. (1994). 'So you did what you wanted then': Discourse analysis, personal agency and psychotherapy. *Journal of Community and Applied Social Psychology, 4*, 261–273.

O'Reilly, M. (2008). What value is there in children's talk? Investigating family therapists' interruptions of parents and children during the therapeutic process. *Journal of Pragmatics, 40*, 507–524.
Päivinen, H., Holma, J., Karvonen, A., Kykyri, V.-L., Tsatsihvili, V., Kaartinen, J., et al. (2016). Affective arousal during blaming in couple therapy: Combining analyses of verbal discourse and physiological responses in two case studies. *Contemporary Family Therapy, 38*(4), 373–384.
Parker, I. (1994). Reflexive research and the grounding of analysis: Social psychology and the 'psy complex. *Journal of Community and Applied Social Psychology, 4*, 239–252.
Parker, I. (Ed.). (1999). *Deconstructing psychotherapy*. London, UK: Sage.
Pärtanen, T., Wahlström, J., & Holma, J. (2006). Loss of self-control as excuse in group therapy conversations for intimately violent men. *Community Medicine, 3*(2), 171–183.
Peräkylä, A., Antaki, C., Vehviläinen, S., & Leudar, I. (Eds.). (2008). *Conversation analysis and psychotherapy*. Cambridge: Cambridge University Press.
Peräkylä, A., Henttonen, P., Voutilainen, L., Kahri, M., Stevanovic, M., Sams, M., et al. (2015). Sharing the emotional load: Recipient affiliation calms down the storyteller. *Social Psychology Quarterly, 78*(4), 301–323.
Pulido-Martinez, H. C. (2014). Psy-complex. In T. Teo (Ed.), *Encyclopedia of critical psychology* (pp. 1598–1599). Springer.
Sampson, E. E. (2003). Possessive individualism and the self-contained ideal. In M. Gergen & K. J. Gergen (Eds.), *Social construction: A reader* (pp. 123–128). London, UK: Sage.
Seikkula, J., Karvonen, A., Kykyri, V.-L., Kaartinen, J., & Penttonen, M. (2015). The embodied attunement of therapists and a couple within dialogical psychotherapy: An introduction to the relational mind project. *Family Process, 54*(4), 703–715.
Seilonen, M. L., Wahlström, J., & Aaltonen, J. (2012). Agency displays on stories of drunk driving: Subjectivity, authorship and reflectivity. *Counselling Psychology Quarterly, 25*(4), 347–360.
Sévon, E. (2011). 'My life has changed but his life hasn't': Making sense of the gendering of parenthood during the transition to motherhood. *Feminism and Psychology, 22*(1), 60–80.
Shotter, J. (1993). *Conversational realities*. London, UK: Sage.
Stancombe, J., & White, S. (2005). Cause and responsibility: Towards an interactional understanding of blaming and 'neutrality' in family therapy. *Journal of Family Therapy, 27*(4), 330–351.

Strong, T., Busch, R., & Couture, S. (2008). Conversational evidence in therapeutic dialogue. *Journal of Marital and Family Therapy, 34*(3), 388–405.
Suoninen, E., & Wahlström, J. (2009). Interactional positions and the production of identities: Negotiating fatherhood in family therapy talk. *Communication & Medicine, 6*(2), 199–209.
Sutherland, O., & Strong, T. (2011). Therapeutic collaboration: A conversation analysis of constructionist therapy. *Journal of Family Therapy, 33*, 256–278.
Tomicic, A., Martinez, C., & Krause, M. (2014). The sound of change: A study of psychotherapeutic process embodied in vocal expression. Laura Rice's ideas revisited. *Psychotherapy Research, 25*(2), 263–276.
Törrönen, J. (2001). The concept of subject position in empirical social research. *Journal for the Theory of Social Behaviour, 31*(3), 313–329.
Voutiläinen, L., Henttonen, P., Kahri, M., Kivioja, M., Ravaja, N., Sams, M., et al. (2014). Affective stance, ambivalence, and psychophysiological responses during conversational storytelling. *Journal of Pragmatics, 68*, 1–24.
Wahlström, J. (2006). The narrative metaphor and the quest for integration in psychotherapy. In E. O'Leary & M. Murphy (Eds.), *New approaches to integration in psychotherapy* (pp. 38–49). London, UK: Routledge.
Weiste, A., & Peräkylä, A. (2014). Prosody and empathic communication in psychotherapy interaction. *Psychotherapy Research, 24*(6), 687–701.
Wetherell, M. (2015). Trends in the turn to affect: A social psychological critique. *Body & Society, 21*(2), 139–166.

4

The Alliance as a Discursive Achievement: A Conversation Analytical Perspective

Adam O. Horvath and Peter Muntigl

Much of the traditional empirical research on therapy prioritizes the study of variables formulated at high levels of abstraction: Active elements of therapy process are conceptualized either as some aggregate qualities of the therapist (e.g., warmth, genuineness, congruence, and alike), attributes of complex therapists' initiated strategies (e.g., the quality of in vivo experiences, the impact of the homework assignments, the value of interpretation or insight, etc.), or as the result of some underlying, but not directly observable, summed relational dynamics such as transference/countertransference, quality of empathy, and so on. The data collected under the influence of this paradigm are numerical or qualitative measures of the observed or reported occurrence of these variables "as such." By "as such" we mean that

A. O. Horvath (✉)
Simon Fraser University, Burnaby, BC, Canada

University Catolica, Santiago, Chile

P. Muntigl
Simon Fraser University, Burnaby, BC, Canada
e-mail: Peter.Muntigl@UGent.be

O. Smoliak, T. Strong (eds.), *Therapy as Discourse*, The Language of Mental Health,
https://doi.org/10.1007/978-3-319-93067-1_4

the process of *how* these variables were realized is most often either assumed to be homogeneous across observations (therefore of little research interest) or the interactive dialectical process between therapist and client that actualize such data are treated as antecedents of the variable of interest and ignored. In addition, research based on this perspective tends to yield descriptions of the therapy process as unidirectional: the observations are organized from the therapist's perspective. The interactive responsive nature of the clinical reality, the dynamic social interactions through which new meanings and insights are realized and new ways of being in the world are discovered are often overlooked, or parked at the margins. Even when relational issues are the focus of investigation, the active elements are frequently conceptualized as therapist activated. For instance, Rogers' notion of the empathy places it in the Therapist Offered Facilitative Conditions (TOFC) framework (Rogers, 1957). In his theory, as well as most of the discourse on "humanistic" therapies, descriptions of the therapy process are focused on what therapists have to offer, his or her personal qualities (e.g., genuineness, presence, etc. (Geller & Greenberg, 2002), and how therapists overcome obstacles and challenges presented by clients, rather than the explication of therapy as a dynamically evolving interactive event.

On the one hand, using abstract, conceptually anchored variables in therapy research offers the obvious advantage of generalizability and replicability of the results. What is observed is assumed to be an [imperfect] actualization of an ideal concept of the variable, thus the results can be abstracted from much of the contextual elements in which it was generated. In this framework the data are summed over many instantiations and become more portable and generalizable in contrast to observations made closer to the phenomenological level—which are more grounded and delimited in the circumstances that generated them. In these research designs, deviations between the actual, observed, realizations and the abstract definition of the variables are either ignored or assigned to the "error term" statistically. Alternatively, the differences between the abstract/conceptual version of the event and what is observed in practice are accounted for as the quality of the variable in the particular instance (e.g., quality/appropriateness of interpretation, level of empathic response, treatment fidelity, etc.). The conceptual/abstract variable stands for an aggregate or class of events or qualities, and the relationships among such aggregate classes can be accurately evaluated statistically.

On the other hand, what is gained through the process of abstraction and categorization of what is essentially an interactive process, are purchased at the cost of limiting what researchers can discover about what makes therapy effective. As Stiles (1988) pointed out, even if we can identify therapeutically active and beneficial variables, such as an efficacious strategy, or a positive relational stance, studying these events "as such" has limited clinical utility: In therapy, examining a strategy apart from the specific context in which it is used will tell you only a part of its therapeutic potential. Increasing the dosage of a "good thing" does not necessarily produce better results (Stiles, Honos-Web, & Surko, 1998). It is, rather, a matter of appropriate responsivity,[1] doing the "right thing" (strategy) at the right time, responding according to the client's needs and resources (Ribeiro et al., 2014; Stiles, 2011; Stiles et al., 1998; Stiles & Horvath, 2017). Research treating interventions or relational elements as "pre-packaged goods" without carefully examining how they are developed, shaped interactively, and made to do therapeutic work in the local context, misses a vital piece which is necessary to get a fuller understanding of how therapy works.

Our research program is designed to complement these more traditional approaches of research by focusing on the exploration of the interactional, conversational praxis of therapy. We start from the basic premise that all forms of psychotherapies, regardless of the particular theoretical framework that underpins the treatment are, at the core, discursive. Psychotherapy inevitably involves some kind of engagement and interaction between a client(s) and a help provider. And this engagement is essentially dialogical in nature involving the negotiation of shared meanings, common goals, and ways to make progress toward these common goals. From this perspective, the differences between treatments that are identified as discursive therapies (e.g., narrative (White, 2007) and those that usually are not labeled as such (e.g., psychoanalysis) refer to the theoretical assumptions with respect to the mechanisms of change but, in each case, the *process of therapy*, what actually happens during treatment is, universally, a series of discursive engagements.

We use Conversation Analysis (CA) as a preferred methodological framework for our investigations. CA treats discourse as a form of social (inter)action in terms of how participants organize their vocal/verbal and

[1] We use the term "appropriate" as Stiles and Horvath (2017) do, to indicate a process of sensitive engagement.

bodily conduct (Peräkylä, 2008; Sidnell & Stivers, 2013), rather than the means of communicating intents pre-formed in our brains. Discursive practices, including therapy, are organized through action sequences and turn-taking resources. It is by way of this sequential organization of our words and grammatical selections and the use of prosody and bodily movements that permit us to make sense of the *other*, negotiate meanings, create social relationships, and "get things done" interactively. Using this approach, we feel, has enabled us to look at therapy processes as a specialized discursive praxis that unfolds, turn by turn, as the participants strive to develop new meanings, position themselves differently in their relationships, and become mutually shaped through each other's actions.

The kind of detailed examination of social interaction afforded by the CA approach is, by its nature, necessarily context dependent. To provide a coherent focus for our research program, we chose to concentrate on aspects of therapy that are recognized as common elements shared by diverse treatments. One of the most obvious such important shared features is that the client and therapist need to develop some level of consensus about the specific aims of the therapy and agree on the things that can be done in therapy to make progress toward these goals. These foundational aspects of therapy—along with the personal bonds that the participants form—are collectively labeled as the therapeutic or working alliance. This concept has its origin in the psychodynamic literature (Greenson, 1990; Horvath & Luborsky, 1993; Zetzel, 1956) but was formally proposed as a universal feature in every kind of treatment by Edward Bordin (1979). Bordin suggested that the acts of developing and sustaining the alliance throughout therapy itself generate a substantive contribution to the healing process. Over the last 45 years, the concept of the alliance has generated a great deal of research, yet relatively little work has been done to closely examine how such relational alignments are realized and repaired in various therapy contexts interactively.

Over the last 15 years, we have pursued a programmatic inquiry using the tools and conceptual resources of CA to take a closer look at how the alliance may be discursively and interactionally accomplished. To do so, we have used an already established discursive-interactional vocabulary to examine how relational alignments and affiliation are maintained, sometimes stressed or ruptured and repaired in clinical situations (Muntigl & Horvath, 2014a). Affiliation and alignment are terms we borrow from CA to capture different types of collaboration between interactants (Stivers, Mondada, & Steensig,

2011). Although these terms are not meant to be "equivalents" to terms used in alliance research, they do, in our opinion, partly explicate the alliance from a discursive-interactional viewpoint. Affiliation refers to practices that are pro-social (e.g., agreeing, complying, etc.) or empathic, whereas alignment refers to cooperative actions that work to get a conversational sequence or activity underway (e.g., actions that support someone's discourse role as storyteller; complying with a request to perform an activity). For example, we have examined how some therapeutic practices, such as making a verbal note of a client's non-vocal conduct (e.g., facial expression, gesture, or bodily movement) and raising it as a salient topic of discussion, can work to bring about closer affiliation between therapists and clients, but also can create dramatic shifts in alignment toward the pursuit of other therapeutic-driven business (Muntigl & Horvath, 2014b). We have also explored how head movements such as nods work to re-equilibrate conversations, repair disaffiliation, and move the participants toward closer affiliation (Muntigl, Knight, Horvath, & Watkins, 2012). For this chapter, we examine a session of family therapy to illustrate a selected set of discursive processes through which stresses in the alliance may occur and how these stresses are subsequently ameliorated. In particular, we show how a therapist and family members work together and orient to and negotiate the alliance with the therapist and also re-negotiate relational allegiances between family members through sequential units of conversation.

Methods

Our research draws on data from therapy sessions with real clients. To illustrate our work, in this chapter we will analyze excerpts from a single session conducted by a master therapist (Dr. S. Minuchin).[2] The session was part of teaching the material Dr. Minuchin prepared for the workshop offered to practicing family therapists. Clients who were receiving service from the institution hosting the workshop were recruited and volunteered to receive a consultation from an "expert therapist." Informed consent to video-tape the consultation and to use the material for train-

[2] We have previously published an analysis of this session examining different research questions (Muntigl & Horvath, 2016).

ing and research purposes was obtained from the client and also from the client's regular therapist who was present at the consultation session.

The client "Suzanne"[3] was a single parent in her early 30s. She had two children: a boy 6 years of age (Kenny) and a girl "Marcy" who was 12 at the time of the interview. The boy was in a special day program (for behavioral difficulties) provided by the host agency. The mother has had long-term substance abuse problems and has been on social assistance for much of her life. She has stopped abusing substances for over a year and has been receiving family therapy (with the children) from a therapist provided by the host agency. The plan was for the family to come in as usual for their weekly appointment, but would receive a consultation from Dr. Minuchin instead of their regular session. Suzanne came with her daughter, but left her little boy with a neighbor who had a boy of similar age.

Present in the excerpts: "Suzanne" (adult client), her daughter "Marcy," "Jenny" the client's regular therapist (a psychologist with over 25 years of experience), and Dr. Minuchin. Initial seating arrangements in the consultation room were: Jenny on the left side of the room on a chair, Marcy and Dr. Minuchin on a couch in the center, Suzanne on the right side of the room sitting on a couch close to Minuchin, and directly opposite Jenny. The session was video recorded and subsequently transcribed using CA transcription conventions, including prosodic elements and significant non-verbal conduct (Hepburn & Bolden, 2013). Some of the transcribed excerpts are reproduced in this chapter, but we used both the video tapes and the transcriptions in our analysis.

Analysis

For our analysis, we have selected three interactional contexts that we feel are exemplary in demonstrating how alliances are forged in family therapy: (1) *diffusing tension and building alliance*, (2) *strengthening "within family" alliances*[4], and (3) *balancing support versus autonomy.*

[3] Pseudonyms are used, and some potentially identifiable material has been altered to protect the privacy of the individuals involved.

[4] To disambiguate the terminology between therapist-client alliances and the realignment and strengthening of relationships between clients, subsequently we shall use the term "allegiance(s)" to

For the first, we show the interactional practices through which the alliance between a therapist and client becomes locally ruptured and then repaired. In the second, we examine how a family therapist discursively works to build a productive allegiance between a mother and daughter, one in which both have a mutual understanding and agreement on family structural relations. And, finally, in the third, we explore how alliance building may run counter to constructing autonomy and authority and how a family therapist works with the clients to balance these therapeutic requirements through specific discursive practices.

Diffusing Tension and Building Alliance

When a family therapist's utterance disaffiliates with a client (or vice versa),[5] it may create tension between these persons and may, momentarily, negatively impact on the degree of social rapport between them. Further, utterances may only indirectly work to disaffiliate, alongside the more central action that the utterance is performing; that is, although an utterance may appear to be functioning primarily as a question, there may also be other kinds of discursive work (e.g., blaming or complaining) generated by the action being carried out. This kind of multi-functionality of utterances may call upon respondents to deal with a number of different issues at the same time. For example, a therapist may need to deal with the tension brought about by the disaffiliation at different levels, such as between therapist-client but perhaps also between family members or even between therapists—if more than one therapist is present in the room. In Extract 1, we show how a therapist's utterance creates tension at these different levels, and, further, we show how Minuchin works at re-building relationships between the different participants including the second therapist present.

refer to the later and use "alliance" exclusively to refer to the therapist/client relationship and collaboration. For further clarification of this terminology, see Symonds and Horvath (2004).

[5] For example, when disagreement, blame, or "acts of defiance" become voiced.

Extract 1

```
01  Jenny:      so (.) maybe we could begin by just, (0.5) <le:tting> me know
02              with what happened with Kenny.=°that >Kenny was planning on
03              coming< toda:y,°
04              (0.6)
05  Jenny:      °an he's not here?°
06              (2.7)
07  Suzanne:    yea:h.
08              (0.6)
09  Suzanne:    um I was- I have to tell you I'm very nervous about today.
10              (1.1)
11  Suzanne:    coming to see you,
      suzanne:              gaze at Minuchin
12              (0.5)
13  Minuchin:   uh- uh so am ↑I:. (.) so [we,   ] .hh so that's good.
14  Suzanne:                             [>yeah<]
15              (0.3)
16  Minuchin:   [w- we are] nervous to↑gether.=
          M&S:  shake hands------------------->
17  Suzanne:    [hh  he   ]                   =°h:heh heh.° oh(.hh)
      suzanne:                          smiles---------------------->

                ((some lines omitted))

18  Suzanne:    Travis, (0.4) I don't think I woulda been able to °get him
19              here today …
20              I w- I ↑woke up, (0.8) °an couldn't-° (0.4) I
21              woke up tryin te manage everybody's life an- (0.4) ↑I just
22              woke up in a really anxious mood.…
23              an I just felt like,
24              >I didn't know which way te go this morning so,<

                ((some lines omitted))

25  Minuchin:   you ↑know Jenny, s-something. (0.6) I think that (0.4)
     minuchin:  gaze at Jenny------------------------------------------->
26              actually,(0.3) may I call you by your first name?=
     minuchin:  ------------>gaze at S-------------------------->
27              =wou[ld you m-]
28  Suzanne:        [Suzanne. ]
29              (0.3)
30  Minuchin:   Suzanne, .hh (.) >I ↑think< (0.9) actually Suzanne, (.)
     minuchin:                        gaze @ Jenny-------------------->
31              did something very nice.
     minuchin:  ---------------------->
32              (1.2)
33  Minuchin:   ↑she decided, (1.5) that Kenny (0.7) was, (1.2)
     minuchin:  continues talking towards Jenny
34              >↑she decided< what is,(0.7) good for Travis.
35              (0.4)
36  Jenny:      °hm.°
37              (1.0)
38  Minuchin:   and ↑she decided that what's good for Kenny toda:y, (0.5)
39              is to be: (0.7)in the regular (0.3) situation.
40              =which he i:s. (0.5) I ↑think its very ↑good.
     minuchin:                            looks b/n S and J
41  Jenny:      °mm hm.°
42              (0.8)
43  Minuchin:   you know, (0.3) instead (.) of responding, (0.7) to your
44              needs or my needs,(0.9) ↑she responded to ↑Kenny's needs.=
```

This extract begins with Jenny, the client's regular therapist, directing a question to the mother, Suzanne (lines 01–03). Through this question, she makes the son's (Kenny) absence a salient topic to be explored in the course of ensuing talk. Jenny's utterance also conveys other actions that create a line of disaffiliation between the participants. To begin, there is an aspect of blame directed at the mother. There was a prior understanding that the mother would bring *both* children to the session, but she arrived only with the daughter. Thus, Suzanne may be viewed as having failed to honor this agreement. Further, Kenny's absence may be seen as reflecting poorly on the client's regular therapist Jenny because she did not deliver the family she promised to have there for Minuchin to work with. Thus, by making it clear that there was an agreement that Travis would be present, Jenny's question may be functioning to defend *herself* and *save face* vis-à-vis Minuchin. We may also note that the son's absence is something that is relevantly reportable, in the first instance, by the parent. By orienting to the *institutional relevance* of the situation in this way (Heritage, 2004), Jenny's talk implies that Suzanne is obligated to inform the other therapists and, by not doing so, the mother's inaction may be viewed as a "misconduct" (Drew, 1998). The blame component of Jenny's talk also performs additional discursive work that promotes further disaffiliation: It puts added pressure on the mother to provide a *satisfactory* explanation of the son's absence. Various turn features illustrate this: "<le:tting> me know" implies that Suzanne is accountable to Jenny; the juxtapositioning of "Kenny was planning to come" with "he's not here" in lines 02–05 creates an implication that Kenny was intending to join them and, thus, his absence constitutes a form of breach.

Jenny's request for information strongly solicits a response or answer (Stivers & Rossano, 2010); that is, it sets up the expectation that Suzanne will respond to the relevant features of the prior action that positioned her as accountable for having committed a breach. Common responses to blame include denial, admission, account, or counter-blame (Buttny, 1993), but, as Buttny has pointed out, response options may be considerably expanded in multi-party participation frameworks. The long delay or silence in line 06 seems to index Suzanne's difficulty in responding, and her confirmatory "yea:h." (line 07) merely acknowledges, but does not answer, Jenny's question. Moreover, her extended response in lines 09–11 seems to stray further from the topic of the son's absence. Although she begins her turn with what might appear as an account in progress ("um I was-"), she quickly *self-repairs*

(Schegloff, Jefferson, & Sacks, 1977) by first drawing attention to the necessity of disclosing something to the therapists ("I have to tell you") and then by using her current emotional state (i.e., her anxiety about coming to see Minuchin) as a discursive resource (and excuse) to shift topic. As well, note that as the mother completes her turn, she directs her gaze at Minuchin, thus making an appeal for Minuchin to take up the next turn. In this way, Suzanne may not only be relieved of the burden of having to answer and account for a certain "misconduct," but it gives another conversational participant a chance to mitigate the mounting anxiety and relationship stress brought on by (1) Jenny's disaffiliative request for an account concerning Kenny's absence and (2) Suzanne's disaffiliative response in which she fails to answer and, instead, implicitly beseeches Minuchin to take up a conversational turn at talk. In this way, Suzanne's utterance functions to disalign with Jenny's initial interactional project of uncovering the "reasons" behind Travis' absence and instead opens up a new line of activity that solicits Minuchin's participation.

Minuchin subsequently complies with Suzanne's implicit non-verbal request by responding to her disclosure of feeling nervous. He does so by first asserting his reciprocating feelings of nervousness ("so am ↑I:.") and, thereafter, by validating their shared emotion ("so that's good. w- we are nervous to↑gether."). Minuchin's response momentarily shifts the topic to "nervousness" and away from "Kenny's absence," thus creating mutual affiliation/alliance around the topic of their shared nervousness. In line 16, Minuchin also shakes hands with Suzanne. Suzanne responds with affiliative laughter (line 17) that claims acceptance of the positive stance realized in Minuchin's prior turn (Schegloff, 2007). Minuchin's attempts at repairing the alliance appear to have been met with some success. In this extract, it is shown how Minuchin uses a disaffiliative episode as an opportunity to form a therapeutic system that helps to build a positive alliance. In Structural Family Therapy (SFT) terms, Minuchin accommodates to the family by professing to also be nervous and works to "join" the family by not only empathizing with but also sharing their "distress."

Later in the conversation, line 18, Suzanne answers Jenny's initial question and thus explicitly orients to issues of blame and accountability by accounting for Kenny's absence. In doing so, she offers confirmation that she breached her parental obligations, but at the same time justifies her conduct by claiming inability ("I don't think I woulda been able to °get him here today"), referencing her anxiety ("woke up in a really anxious mood") and displaying uncertainty (">I didn't know which way te go this morning so,<"). These displays of uncertainty, uneasiness, and low agency have potential negative implications that create a self-deprecating stance: She is not a good mother and the "proof" is that she was unable to bring Kenny to therapy. Research in CA on everyday conversation has shown that self-deprecations are generally followed by two different response types: The first is affiliative, working to strengthen social relations, and consists of disagreeing with the self-deprecation or offering praise, whereas the second is disaffiliative and consists of agreeing with other's negative assessment of self (Pomerantz, 1984).

In his response from lines 25–44, Minuchin performs detailed moral and affiliative work by drawing from a range of interactional resources that orient toward the alliance between himself and Jenny, but also between the therapists (Minuchin and Jenny) and Suzanne. Beginning in line 25, Minuchin directs his talk to the other therapist ("you ↑know Jenny…"), thus momentarily changing the participation framework of the interaction by orienting both physically and verbally to Jenny and away from Suzanne and by making Suzanne a type of *by-stander* to the conversation (Goffman, 1981), someone who is no longer a ratified participant in the conversation and can only *listen*. His subsequent formulation of "I think that … actually," lines 25–26, seems to foretell an upcoming difference of opinion; in fact, the sequential placement of "actually" implies that Minuchin is about to provide a different account of the events surrounding Travis' absence. This shift in the participation framework performs alliance building work in two important ways: First, it allows the therapists to momentarily "join in alliance or coalition" with Jenny (Minuchin, 1974, p. 148), thus repairing the relational damage created by "interrupting" Jenny's original line of inquiry and by recognizing and promoting Jenny as the relevant person to affirm the new framework presented. Second, as will be shown later in the sequence, it positions the therapists as being "in agreement" as to how Suzanne positively dealt with the situation, thus establishing re-affiliation with the mother.

In line 26, Minuchin briefly returns to the "original" participation framework in which Suzanne is a ratified participant by requesting permission to use her first name ("may I call you by your first name?"). Through this move, he works to re-establish an alliance with Suzanne. Subsequently, in line 30 onward, he again resumes his coalition with Jenny by making eye contact with and directing his talk at her. While doing so, he now completes his alternative interpretation of events, as indexed by the term "actually," and then does affiliative work by praising Suzanne's decision not to bring Kenny (">I ↑think< (0.9) actually Suzanne, (.) did something very nice. …"). Thereafter, he orients to and highlights Suzanne's authoritative role of mother/caregiver (">↑she decided< what is, (0.7) good for Kenny."; "you know, (0.3) instead (.) of responding, (0.7) to your needs or my needs, (0.9) ↑she responded to ↑Kenny's needs.=). Note also that Minuchin emphasizes and strengthens his positive assessment through prosodic resources of stress and rising pitch and that Jenny weakly affiliates by offering her acknowledgment (lines 15 and 19). Thus, Minuchin's discursive practices provide Suzanne with an opportunity to re-consider her position vis-à-vis Minuchin's and to consider accepting the agentive and authoritative position that Minuchin is offering her. This strategy also allows Minuchin to perform a face-threatening act (i.e., disagreement with Jenny) in a face-saving and thus affiliative manner: He is actually telling another therapist about how positive the mother's actions were, contrary to what the mother (Suzanne) may have thought. Also, by forming a coalition of alliance between himself and Jenny through the altered participation framework, Minuchin not only helps to smooth over what might be considered a difference in views between the therapists but also gives Jenny the opportunity to make a display of shifting perspectives and thus affiliating with this new agentive position for the mother. As can be recalled, from Jenny's initial perspective, Suzanne had undergone a breach by not bringing Travis. But from Minuchin's viewpoint, Suzanne was demonstrating authority, an action that deserves praise.

Strengthening "Within Family" Allegiances

One of the initial contexts for family therapy involves a disalignment in perspectives regarding family role relationships. Whereas the parents may show difficulty in adopting certain age and stage-appropriate "executive" roles vis-à-vis their children, the children, in turn, may be uncertain about which roles they may assume and how these may work to complement parental roles. To achieve good allegiances between family members, it becomes necessary that clarity and endorsement of respective roles be realized. One of the main therapeutic objectives in SFT is achieving mutual understanding and agreement on family roles. Consider Extract 2, in which Minuchin initiates a dialogue with the mother and daughter to gain consensus on role relationships and tasks. Just previously, Minuchin wondered whether the family situation sometimes led Marcy to conduct herself in ways more typical of an 18 years old (i.e., a grown-up) and, moreover, that Marcy's resistance to parental authority may be related to that. This was then followed by Suzanne reflecting on the difficult life she had growing up and if that bore any relation to Marcy's life and her being 12 years old.

Extract 2: [14:55]

```
Suzanne:     I don't know.=↑I'm not making any sense. [ I-   I'm] (.)
Minuchin:                                             [you make,]
  suzanne:   gaze moves up, hands to head, adjusts herself in the seat
 minuchin:                                    reaches out and touches B's arm
Suzanne:     I don't=[know.=I-    ]
Minuchin:            [(you rilly)] make, you make a lot of sense [to me:.
Suzanne:                                                           [°I don't
             know.°
             (0.8)
Minuchin:    you make a lot of sense to me.
             (0.4)
Minuchin:    >uh.< (0.5) does she make↑ sense to you.
             (1.1)
Marcy:       yeah.
             (1.3)
Minuchin:    but ↑mo:m doesn't feel frequently that she has, (0.5) the
             ri:ght, (1.4) to, (1.2) to make ru:les for you.=is that true?
             (0.5)
Marcy:       we:ll:.
             (0.9)
Marcy:       I think she has the right to make rules for me,=>but I jus<
             don't like the rules she makes.
             (0.9)
Minuchin:    but you know (.) what I:↑ (0.5) hea:r, (0.5) is that mo:m
             feels very frequently, (0.6) that she needs (.) to, (0.8)
             ↑apologize to you for being your ↑mom.
             (0.8)
Minuchin:    is that true.
             (0.8)
Minuchin:    does she do that?
             (0.5)
Marcy:       mm hm.
    marcy:   multiple shallow nods
             (1.7)
Minuchin:    an what do you think.
             (1.3)

             ((lines omitted))

Marcy:       I:, (0.3) ↑I used to think it was, (0.3) we:ll, I still do
             think >some of the times it's< ↑my fault.=[but I jus] can't
Minuchin:                                               [ yea:h. ]
    marcy:                                              shakes head
Marcy:       bring myself to say I'm ↑sorry=ri:ght?=
Minuchin:    =yea:h. (0.6) so you have- (.) both of you have a problem.
             (1.3) °both of you have a problem because,° (1.3) you need,
             (1.0) a mom that can give you, (0.8) that can be a mom, (.)
             who is not apologizing.
             (1.1)
Minuchin:    an (0.5) <you don't fee:l> you have the <ri:ght sometimes,>
             (1.7) to be ↑it. (1.2) Kar- (.) uh u:h, (0.4) Marcy's mom? (.)
             it's- it's an interesting thing.
```

At the beginning of this extract, Suzanne makes numerous displays of uncertainty ("I don't know."; "↑I'm not making any sense.") and nonverbal displays of discomfort such as shifting around in her seat and placing her hands to her head. From the daughter's perspective, this may be seen as a confirmation of "weakness" in which the mother appears uncertain, as someone who is unable to confidently appropriate a position of epistemic authority. It is likely for this reason that Minuchin immediately aligns with the mother by showing strong endorsement of the mother's epistemic status and her ability to make perfect sense to others ("you make a lot of sense to me:."). Minuchin also strongly affiliates with Suzanne by using intensifiers such as "rilly" and "a lot of" and by touching her arm during a brief moment of distress and uncertainty. He then repeats his endorsement of Suzanne's ability to make sense and then asks Marcy whether she is of the same opinion. Through this move, Minuchin works to gain Marcy's endorsement of her mother as someone with entitlements to knowledge and experience and as someone whose talk is transparent and logical. When Marcy voices agreement in line 12, Minuchin then in lines 14–15 leverages her response in order to draw Marcy's attention to the implied paradox of having parental authority, while at the same time not having rights to make rules for your children. Minuchin casts this viewpoint from the mother's perspective ("but ↑mo:m doesn't feel frequently that…"), which works to downgrade his own epistemic position (i.e., it is the mother that claims this, not Minuchin), but he also cedes epistemic rights to Marcy by giving her the opportunity to respond to the mother's feelings ("is that true?"). Minuchin's use of "frequently"—see also line 23—also works as a shield against the possible inference that Minuchin is being critical of Suzanne's performance as mother; that is, although Suzanne frequently does not enact her parental authority, she does at times do so. In this way, Minuchin works to create a balance between having to discuss the mother's difficulty in adopting a parental role with Marcy, while at the same time not leaving the impression that the mother is unable to exert authority. By way of response, Marcy makes partial concessions to the mother's viewpoint ("I think she has the right to make rules for me,=>but…"), but then continues by voicing disagreement about the content of the rules ("I jus< don't like the rules she makes."). Thus, by first forming a strong alignment with the mother to support her role as someone who has legitimate parental authority and then getting Marcy to affiliate with this position, Minuchin has taken first steps in achieving a new allegiance between the family members. This is one in which the mother's actions begin to "make sense" from the reference point of the daughter.

Later, in lines 22–28, Minuchin again tries to solicit the daughter's agreement on what appears to be a dysfunctional structural hierarchy between the parent and child. He prefaces his turn with an evidential expression ("what I: ↑ (0.5) hea:r") that displays his lesser access and knowledge about what Marcy's mother is actually feeling. Thus, the ensuing claim that the mother needs to apologize to Marcy when acting like a parental authority is put on record as based on hearsay and is thus presented as a possibility that seeks confirmation from Marcy. Note that Minuchin uses the term "frequently," which again—as in line 14—works subtly to endorse the mother's parental role as someone who is able to enact authority. Also, Minuchin's choice of the word "need" as in ("she needs (.) to, ↑apologize…") further suggests that the mother may be facing certain "familial" obstacles preventing her from enacting control (e.g., she may feel she *needs* to apologize in order to maintain an affiliative mother-daughter relationship) and, by implication, changing the present mother-daughter patterns of communication may facilitate an improved way of relating. This epistemically downgraded turn design allows Marcy to not only confirm the veracity of this claim, but to also reflect and elaborate on the reasons why this may be so. Although Marcy does not immediately respond, she does, after a couple of confirmation-seeking prompts, provide verbal and non-verbal affiliation. After having gained Marcy's confirmation, Minuchin proceeds to probe into the reasons why the mother may have trouble taking up authority by asking for Marcy's opinion ("an wh<u>at</u> do you t<u>hi</u>nk."). What follows is a concession in which Marcy takes some responsibility for the family dynamics (lines 34–37); that is, she concedes that she sometimes may be at fault (rather than her mother, thus absolving the mother of the need to apologize) but is unable to apologize to her mother. With this concession, Minuchin has managed to move the family a bit closer to achieving mutual understanding on the problem and to forming the preconditions for forging a different allegiance in which the mother and daughter may begin to construct their relationship in a more productive way.

From line 38 onward, Minuchin begins to summarize the family's dilemma, framing it as an issue of joint responsibility reinforced by the repeated use of "both of you" (lines 38–39): Marcy needs a parental figure who does not apologize for exercising her entitled authority, and Suzanne does not feel entitled to take up this authoritative position. Then, in line 45, Minuchin frames the dilemma as a puzzle ("it's- it's an interesting thing"), which does a range of epistemic work: It implies that Minuchin does not have special insight into why this problem occurs, and consequently, he declines responsibility to deliver a solution; it suggests that further reflection and exploration may allow the family to "solve the puzzle" and create a more positive relationship; and it operates as a *fishing device* (Pomerantz, 1980), because it targets the family members' personal epistemic domains to which they may display greater rights and access.

Balancing Support Versus Autonomy

It is not uncommon for clients to experience and display emotional distress during a session. These displays have therapeutic significance not only because they provide access into the client's emotional experiences, but because they provide opportunities for affiliation and empathy and thus the potential for forging a strong alliance between the participants. There are cases in family therapy, however, where displays of upset may create certain therapeutic dilemmas: On the one hand, distress calls for support from the group, but this support may also undermine the upset person's autonomy, thus making them appear "needy" and unable to take control of the situation. In Extract 3, it is shown how Minuchin is able to balance the needs of support versus autonomy in a context where Suzanne becomes emotionally distressed. Although Minuchin offers Suzanne support, he is careful not to impinge on her autonomy, making her look weak in the eyes of her daughter, and to resist attempts by others to undercut the mother's authority.

Extract 3: [17:00]

```
01   Suzanne:    I think >in a< ↑wa:y uh, (1.7) I find it ha:rd when (.) I have
       suzanne:                gaze up
02               to put my foot down with her,=because, .hh (.) it is such a
03               ↑fi:ght. (0.8) it is such a ↑fi:ght.
04   Minuchin:   well but [it's e-   ]
05   Suzanne:             [that I- ↑I] I feel like, (.) [ I f::-] uf- the
06   Minuchin:                                          [°yeah.° ]
07   Suzanne:    ↑fe:ar that comes=↑i:n me. (0.3) °is is° is [overwhelming.]
08   Minuchin:                                               [but   what. ]
09               (1.2)
10   Minuchin:   what is the fe:ar.
11               (1.5)
12   Suzanne:    the ↑fear of reJEC↑tion=the fear of her telling me .hh to-
13               (1.4)
       suzanne:  opens mouth, circular motion with head
14   Minuchin:   so you- you need her to love you euh?
15               (0.4)
16   Suzanne:    hhhhhhh
       suzanne:  smile, double nod
17               (1.5)
       suzanne:  looks @ Minuchin, nod
18   Minuchin:   °e-° that's very important.
19               (0.3)
20   Minuchin:   you're very important to your mom.
      minuchin:  directs talk to Marcy
21               (2.6)
22   Minuchin:   it is very important that you [show,
23   Suzanne:                                  [°snih°
24               (0.7)
25   Minuchin:   [love an (        )  ] an [   app]rove.
26               [~excuse me, eh heh~]     [>yep.<]
27               (0.8)
28   Minuchin:   °yeah.°
29               (1.7)
30   Minuchin:   e- is that, (0.5) is that very heavy on y[ou.]
31   Suzanne:                                             [hh ] ~u:h excuse me
32               Jenny. thanks~
33               (2.0)
       suzanne:  gets up, moves off camera
34   Suzanne:    °snih° [~it was really ↑ha:rd] for me to say that.~
35   Jenny:             [    there's ti-      ]
       suzanne:  off camera------------------------------------------>
36               (0.7)
37   Minuchin:   °no↓ no no. [c'm in here.° let's just-
      minuchin:  gestures for S to return
38   Jenny:                  [come on Sue. here's some tissues. (        )
39               (1.0)
         Marcy:  reaches to pass tissue box, that is beside her, to her crying
                 mother, who is standing searching for tissues
40   Minuchin:   ↑NO: no no no.=let- (.) let her take it. (0.4) °let her take
41               it.°
```

At the beginning of this extract, Suzanne is discussing the difficulties she is having with Marcy (lines 01–07). She finds it hard "to put my foot down" and that "it is s̲u̲ch a ↑f̲i̲:ght." She then, in line 07, reveals her emotional state in these situations as one of overwhelming fear. Following a prompt by Minuchin in line 10, in which he attempts to elicit more talk about the fear (for elicitation practices, see Muntigl & Hadic Zabala, 2008), Suzanne complies by naming "the ↑fear of reJEC↑tion" and then begins to verbalize what Marcy may say to her in these contexts but cuts it off (line 12). She does, however, provide Minuchin with non-verbal access of what Marcy bodily performs through a *reenactment* (Sidnell, 2006), in which Suzanne mimics the facial and head movements during which Marcy may be rejecting her. After having conveyed her emotional assessment of typical situations involving her daughter, Minuchin proceeds to utter a *formulation* (Antaki, 2008), that provides the upshot of Suzanne's fear of rejection, "so you- you need her to love you euh?", and that underscores how important it is for the mother and daughter to maintain a close, affectionate relationship. It is at this point that Suzanne begins to shows signs of distress: She produces a pronounced sigh (line 16), then begins to sniff (line 23), which is followed in line 26 by an apology that is delivered in a *tremulous voice* (Hepburn & Potter, 2007) and, finally, another apology with tremulous voice followed by her moving off camera (line 33). During this time, Minuchin repeatedly points out the significance of Suzanne's emotional self-disclosure to Marcy—"you're very important to your mom." (line 20); "it is very important that you show, love an ( ) an approve." (lines 22 & 25)—and later, in line 30, attempts to solicit her feelings concerning the important role she plays in her mom's life.

Still showing signs of deep distress, Suzanne concedes in line 34 that her prior self-disclosure was difficult and, in would seem, painful ("°snih° ~it was really ↑ha:rd for me to say that.~"). Jenny then produces an overlapping affiliative move of offering Suzanne some tissues (line 35), which is followed by Minuchin's attempt to get Suzanne to return to her seat (line 37) and Jenny's overlapping utterance that repeats her offer, but this time in full. Following this, in line 39, Marcy reaches for the tissue box in an attempt to hand them over to Suzanne. Minuchin is then quick to reject and block Marcy's offer, demanding that Suzanne take the tissues herself ("let her take it. (0.4) °let her take it.°"). From a Structural Family Therapy perspective, the unfolding sequence is an "enactment" of the family's problematic tendency to reverse mother/daughter roles under stressful conditions: In offering the tissue box to her mother, Suzanne is placed in a role of dependency in which her daughter provides for her. This role relationship is what Minuchin has been trying to reverse through his interactions with the family and that would explain why he resists Marcy's attempt so vigorously. In doing so, Minuchin implies that Suzanne is able to fend for herself, that she can recover from distressing situations. Thus, although Marcy's gesture on the surface does have an affiliative quality, it does so at the expense of undermining Suzanne's position as an agentic and autonomous parental authority.

Conclusions

The analyses above provide examples of the ways we approach analyzing therapy process using CA. Examining therapy as an interactive phenomena unfolding in language can help to illuminate the discursive elements that dynamically realize relational structures in therapy. For example, the analyses allow us to follow, turn by turn, how a potentially disruptive interaction can be worked through to establish a pivotal alignment with the parent and, at the same time, challenge her traditional self-critical defensive response and generate creative novel alternatives to explore. CA methods enable us to identify the specific conversational resources used and the way these resources are sequenced and timed to create an opportunity in the discourse for the client to move from the position of "failure" to "success," from powerlessness to agentic identity. The first excerpt also provides an opportunity to observe how the use of timing, phrasing, emphases, and direction of turns in the conversation can realize multiple therapeutic objectives: Prevent potential disaffiliation between the two therapists, foreclose the danger of the parent defensively disenfranchising herself (which is her previous, pathogenic, pattern), and at the same time establish a preferred relational position with both the other therapist (Jenny) and the client.

The detailed "microscopic" attention to conversational elements also enables us to track how "appropriate responsiveness," doing the right thing at the right time (Stiles & Horvath, 2017), is realized in a clinical situation: In the second example, the therapist again has to deal with the mother's self-deprecating stance, but this time he leverages the strong alliance developed earlier in the interview with the daughter (Marcy) to re-align the relationship between mother and child. Asking Marcy to align with Minuchin's assertion of the "right moral order" in the family, in some sense, undermines her own rebellious position with her mother. The analysis provides us with a better understanding of how phrasing and timing creates a "safe place" for Marcy to explore the dynamics between her and mum in a non-defensive way. In SFT the goal is to frame the difficulties the system encounters as a shared struggle to achieve functional roles within the family. In Excerpt #2 we were able to explore an example of the discursive work that realizes this goal: The therapist refers to the ongoing conflict as an "interesting thing." The positioning of the issue as "interesting" has a potentially positive connotation which is juxtapositioned with the use of the term "problem" that "you" (plural) have. The use of "problem" eliminates culpability, and at the same time "you" (plural) re-emphasizes the theme of mutuality, and suggeststs that the challenge the family faces is a relational issue. The CA analysis draws attention to how this shift from blame to the need to fulfill both mothers' and child's needs is realized sequentially and interactively The sequential examination of the communicative turns allows to explicate the nuanced ways the therapist and the clients work discursively to shape new alignments and search for a "new" vision of what is happening between mother and child. In SFT terms Minuchin is re-structuring the family, introducing a hierarchical moral order with parents exercising executive functions and children benefiting from the protection and age-appropriate autonomy such structure provides. We believe that our CA analysis provides the critical window on the dynamic responsivity involved in the implementation of his therapeutic objectives. Importantly, this perspective provides the conceptual framework and analytic tools to explicate how the therapeutic process involves attentive work on relational alignments not only between therapist and clients but between clients themselves.

As we noted in the beginning of this essay, our overall goal is to gain a clearer understanding of how various aspects of the alliance are built, maintained, and made effective in therapy. Examining therapy discourse sequentially in fine-grained detail has provided us with a clearer view of how the relational aspects of treatment are developed interactively, how these alliances partner with various therapeutic objectives and realize forward movement in treatment. The extracts we provided were drawn from a family therapy session. Exploring data from a multi-person context has provided particularly rich opportunities to analyze the way discourse works to not only realize therapeutic objectives between therapist and clients individually, but also re-shape allegiances through selecting participants and structuring the flow of conversation. However, the analytic methods and perspectives we demonstrated are equally applicable and useful to explicate the discursive processes that are at the core of individual psychotherapy irrespective of the theoretical orientation guiding the process (Buchholtz & Kächele, 2017). We believe that, from a broader perspective, research on the essentially discursive, interactive nature of psychotherapy at this detailed level provides a needed compliment to quantitative psychotherapy research.

References

Antaki, C. (2008). Formulations in psychotherapy. In A. Peräkylä, C. Antaki, S. Vehviläinen, & I. Leudar (Eds.), *Conversation analysis and psychotherapy* (pp. 26–42). Cambridge: Cambridge University Press.

Bordin, E. S. (1979). The generalizability of the psychoanalytic concept of the working alliance. *Psychotherapy: Theory, Research & Practice, 16*(3), 252–260. https://doi.org/10.1037/h0085885

Buchholtz, M. B., & Kächele, H. (2017). From turn-by-turn to larger chunks of talk: An exploratory study in psychotherapeutic micro-processes using conversation analysis. *Research in Psychotherapy: Psychopathology, Process and Outcome, 20*, 161–178.

Buttny, R. (1993). *Social accountability in communication*. London: Sage.

Drew, P. (1998). Complaints about transgressions and misconduct. *Research on Language and Social Interaction, 31*, 295–325.

Geller, S. M., & Greenberg, L. S. (2002). Therapeutic presence: Therapists' experience of presence in the psychotherapy encounter. *Person-Centered and Experiential Psychotherapies, 1*(1–2), 71–86.

Goffman, E. (1981). Footing. In E. Goffman (Ed.), *Forms of talk* (pp. 124–159). Oxford: Basil Blackwell.

Greenson, R. R. (1990). The working alliance and the transference neurosis. In A. H. Esman & A. H. Esman (Eds.), *Essential papers on transference* (pp. 150–171). New York, NY: New York University Press.

Hepburn, A., & Bolden, G. (2013). The conversation analytic approach to transcription. In J. Sidnell & T. Stivers (Eds.), *The handbook of conversation analysis* (pp. 57–76). Chichester, UK: Wiley-Blackwell.

Hepburn, A., & Potter, J. (2007). Crying receipts: Time, empathy, and institutional practice. *Research on Language and Social Interaction, 40*, 89–116.

Heritage, J. (2004). Conversation analysis and institutional talk: Analyzing data. In D. Silverman (Ed.), *Qualitative research: Theory, method and practice* (2nd ed., pp. 222–245). London: Sage.

Horvath, A. O., & Luborsky, L. (1993). The role of the therapeutic alliance in psychotherapy. *Journal of Consulting and Clinical Psychology, 61*, 561–573.

Minuchin, S. (1974). *Families & family therapy*. Cambridge, MA: Harvard University Press.

Muntigl, P., & Hadic Zabala, L. (2008). Expandable answers: How clients get prompted to say more during psychotherapy. *Research on Language and Social Interaction, 41*(2), 187–226.

Muntigl, P., & Horvath, A. O. (2014a). The therapeutic relationship in action: How therapists and clients co-manage relational disaffiliation. *Psychotherapy Research*. https://doi.org/10.1080/10503307.2013.807525

Muntigl, P., & Horvath, A. O. (2014b). "I can see some sadness in your eyes": When experiential therapists notice a client's affectual display. *Research on Language and Social Interaction, 47*(2), 89–108.

Muntigl, P., & Horvath, A. O. (2016). A conversation analytic study of building and repairing the alliance in family therapy. *Journal of Family Therapy, 38*(1), 102–119. https://doi.org/10.1111/1467-6427.12109

Muntigl, P., Knight, N., Horvath, A. O., & Watkins, A. (2012). Client affectual stance and therapist-client affiliation: A view from grammar and social interaction. *Research in Psychotherapy: Psychopathology, Process and Outcome, 15*(2), 117–130.

Peräkylä, A. (2008). *Conversation analysis and psychotherapy/edited by Anssi Peräkylä … [et al.]* (A. Peräkylä, Trans.). Cambridge: Cambridge University Press.

Pomerantz, A. (1980). Telling my side: "Limited access" as a "fishing" device. *Sociological Inquiry, 50*, 186–198.

Pomerantz, A. (1984). Agreeing and disagreeing with assessment: Some features of preferred/dispreferred turn shapes. In J. Atkinson & J. Heritage (Eds.), *Structures of social action: Studies in conversation analysis* (pp. 57–101). Cambridge: Cambridge University Press.

Ribeiro, A. P., Ribeiro, E., Loura, J., Gonçalves, M. M., Stiles, W. B., Horvath, A. O., et al. (2014). Therapeutic collaboration and resistance: Describing the nature and quality of the therapeutic relationship within ambivalence events using the Therapeutic Collaboration Coding System. *Psychotherapy Research, 24*(3), 346–359. https://doi.org/10.1080/10503307.2013.856042

Rogers, C. R. (1957). The necessary and sufficient conditions of therapeutic personality change. *Journal of Consulting and Clinical Psychology, 22*, 95–103.

Schegloff, E. A. (2007). *Sequence organization in interaction: A primer in conversation analysis*. Cambridge: Cambridge University Press.

Schegloff, E. A., Jefferson, G., & Sacks, H. (1977). The preference for self-correction in the organization of repair in conversation. *Language, 53*, 361–382.

Sidnell, J. (2006). Coordinating gesture, talk, and gaze in reenactments. *Research on Language and Social Interaction, 39*(4), 377–409.

Sidnell, J., & Stivers, T. (Eds.). (2013). *The handbook of conversation analysis*. Oxford, UK: Wiley-Blackwell.

Stiles, W. B. (1988). Psychotherapy process-outcome relations may be misleading. *Psychotherapy: Theory, Research, Practice and Training, 25*, 27–35.

Stiles, W. B. (2011). Coming to terms. *Psychotherapy Research, 21*(4), 367–384.

Stiles, W. B., Honos-Web, L., & Surko, M. (1998). Responsiveness in psychotherapy. *Clinical Psychology: Science and Practice, 5*, 439–458.

Stiles, W. B., & Horvath, A. O. (2017). Appropriate responsiveness as a contribution to therapist effects. In L. G. Castonguay & C. E. Hill (Eds.), *Therapist effects: Toward understanding how and why some therapists are better than others* (pp. 71–84). Washington, DC: APA Books.

Stivers, T., Mondada, L., & Steensig, J. (2011). Knowledge, morality and affiliation in social interaction. In T. Stivers, L. Mondada, & J. Steensig (Eds.), *The morality of knowledge in conversation* (pp. 3–24). Cambridge: Cambridge University Press.

Stivers, T., & Rossano, F. (2010). Mobilizing response. *Research on Language and Social Interaction, 43*, 3–31.

Symonds, B. D., & Horvath, A. O. (2004). Optimizing the alliance in couple therapy. *Family Process, 43*(4), 443–455.

White, M. (2007). *Maps of narrative practice*. New York, NY: W. W. Norton & Co.

Zetzel, E. R. (1956). Current concepts of transference. *International Journal of Psychoanalysis, 37*, 369–376.

5

Discursive Therapies as Institutional Discourse

Gale Miller

I offer an approach to discursive therapies as institutional discourse in this paper. Discursive therapies are relatively new developments in the therapy world (Lock & Strong, 2012). They mirror discursive trends in philosophy and the social sciences over the past century (Hacker, 2013; Weinberg, 2008). Discursively oriented philosophers and social scientists treat people's uses of language as creative activities that are comparable to their other—seemingly non-discursive—activities, such as building bridges, cooking meals, or doing surgery. This orientation is basic to social constructionist perspectives in philosophy, the social sciences, and therapy (Holstein & Gubrium, 2008; Lock & Strong, 2010). The perspectives consider how people's senses of themselves and their worlds emerge as they interact with each other.

Strong and Lock (2005) depict discursive therapy interactions as collaborative conversations concerned with what clients want and the resources available to clients in achieving their preferred futures.

G. Miller (✉)
Department of Social and Cultural Sciences, Marquette University, Milwaukee, WI, USA
e-mail: gale.miller@marquette.edu

O. Smoliak, T. Strong (eds.), *Therapy as Discourse*, The Language of Mental Health,
https://doi.org/10.1007/978-3-319-93067-1_5

Discursive therapy interactions are negotiations about what appear to be the facts of clients' lives and how else those seeming facts might be understood. Similar to discursively oriented philosophers and social scientists, discursive therapists treat social interactions as producing conditions for transforming persons' senses of social reality (Anderson & Gehart, 2007; Miller & McKergow, 2012; White, 2007). Discursive therapies might be characterized as forms of applied social constructionism designed to foster such transformations.

Some readers might argue that the word *institution* does not apply to discursive therapy practices or relationships. The term is sometimes used to characterize rigid and hierarchical structures designed to limit people's options, if not fully control them. These readers might add that discursive therapies are designed to produce flexible and cooperative relationships that help clients to see themselves and their lives in new ways. Thus, it is important to be clear about what I mean when I say that discursive therapies form an institutional discourse. I use this term to call attention to the interrelated language and interpretive practices associated with one or more institutional settings (Miller, 1994). Language practices include the ways that participants in institutional settings ask and answer questions, describe the unfolding of events in situations, and elaborate on or counter others' depictions of issues. Interpretive practices are the methods that people use in constructing and assigning meanings to issues emergent in social interactions.

A discourse is a body of resources that people use in making sense of their experiences and managing their lives. In shifting from one discourse to another, people engage different language and interpretive resources that may transform their senses of themselves and their lives. Fostering such shifts is, of course, fundamental to discursive therapy practices. While every approach to discursive therapy is somewhat unique, discursive therapies may be analyzed as institutional discourse because they share fundamental assumptions about the meanings at issue in therapist-client relationships and utilize similar interactional methods in exploring those meanings (Georgaca & Advi, 2009).

Institutional discourses and the settings with which they are associated are interactively linked. Each forms a background for the other. Typical spaces, objects, and activities making up institutional settings are discursive in signaling the sorts of interactional work done by participants in the settings. Institutional settings might be interpreted as preludes to persons' entrance into institutional discourses. Initial discursive signals are transformed into concrete relationships and constructions of social reality as participants negotiate the issues at hand in their interactions. Participants in the interactions may continue to attend to aspects of institutional settings in asserting their preferred orientations. Thus, the institutional discourse of discursive therapies includes both the settings in which the therapies are practiced and the language and assumptions used by participants in the settings.

Backdrop and Organization

Contemporary discursive therapies did not appear full-blown. They emerged in prior supportive environments for developing alternatives to therapy approaches based on the medical model (Ray, 1999). The medical model turns on treating clients' symptoms as caused by underlying conditions that therapists diagnose for their clients. It justifies a moral division of labor in which therapists are experts empowered to direct clients toward professionally approved treatments. The division of labor is moral because it defines how therapist-client interactions *should* be organized (Weakland, 1999). It represents an institutionally preferred social reality for medically oriented therapists. Hughes (1971) characterizes this orientation to professional-client relationships as the traditional North American conception of professionalism.

> Professionals *profess*. They profess to know better than others the nature of certain matters, and to know better than their clients what ails them or their affairs. This is the essence of the professional idea and the professional claim. (Hughes, 1971, p. 375)

Proponents of contemporary discursive therapies have extended and—to varying degrees—transformed their forbearers' innovations in therapy practices. They have repositioned therapists and clients, making their relationships less hierarchical and defining clients as possessing useful knowledge about the future possibilities for clients' lives. Contemporary discursive therapists are also disinclined to search for the underlying causes of their clients' problems or classify clients' problems within fixed categories associated with pre-determined solutions. The therapists do not promise to cure their clients' problems but to support clients' efforts to construct more satisfactory lives for themselves.

These aspects of discursive therapies form a conventional wisdom that discursive therapists advocate to each other and to interested parties outside their community (Tarragona, 2008). It includes claims about what discursive therapists should stand for (e.g., therapist-client relationships as partnerships, valuing multiple perspectives, and being curious about clients' experiences) and against (e.g., diagnosing, pathologizing, or morally judging clients and their problems). A major theme in this conventional wisdom is that therapist-client interactions should be collaborative. This theme is indicative of how clients and therapists are socially constructed in the institutional discourse of discursive therapies. Both are defined as having distinctive competencies and responsibilities in their interactions.

My point is not to criticize discursive therapists for doing what all professional groups do in building shared identities. Rather, it is to say that discursive therapists also profess and that their claims justify discursive therapists' orientations to therapy. The claims constitute an institutionally preferred reality that discursive therapists use in assessing the appropriateness of their own and others' practices. Such claims may become problematic, however, when we shift attention to the practical circumstances associated with diverse therapist-client interactions. The circumstances include the distinctive histories of clients' lives, clients' preferred ways of interacting with their therapists, and the practical contexts of therapy interactions. The latter contexts include insurance company rules, legal regulations, and referring agency expectations to which discursive therapists may be accountable.

One thread in discursive social science research deals with how people manage such contingencies in social interactions. The research explores how people cast practical circumstances as matters of concern. Discursive studies document how people orient to shared values that extend beyond particular interactions while responding to pressing issues that organize particular interactions. The studies also promise to reveal participant competencies that often go unnoticed in everyday assessments and descriptions of social interactions, including assessments and descriptions made by discursive therapists about their interactions with clients.

I extend the themes raised in this and the previous section in the rest of the paper. Three general concerns inform the discussion. The first involves how discursive perspectives in therapy and the social sciences are different but compatible orientations to discursive therapist-client interactions. The second focuses on how discursive therapy discourse organizes therapist-client interactions as practical and moral encounters. The third issue attends to the usefulness of discursively oriented empirical research in describing how social realities are constructed in discursive therapy interactions. I draw from the writings of discursive therapists and researchers, as well as my observations of discursive therapist-client interactions, in the sections that follow. I begin by elaborating on the concept of discursive therapies as institutional discourse and then summarize aspects of three discursive perspectives in the social sciences (ethnomethodology, conversation analysis, and Foucauldian discourse studies). These sections form a background for re-examining the claim that discursive therapist-client relationships are collaborative.

Thinking About Institutional Discourse

Institutional discourses are dynamic sites for the construction of social realities. Social realities emerge as people in interaction depict, interpret, and justify practical responses to issues that they encounter in institutional settings. Socially constructed realities are sustained, modified, and may be displaced by alternative realities as people continue to interact in institutional settings. These possibilities in institutional interactions make the social construction of institutional realities both predictable and unpredictable. The process is predictable because contemporary social institutions are defined by the typical (preferred) terminologies, meanings, and actions taken by persons working within them (Emerson & Messinger, 1977). Institutional interactions that stray too far from preferred patterns risk being deemed illegitimate by participants in institutional settings. Unexpected social realities sometimes emerge in institutional interactions as participants assess the relevance of atypical orientations for particular situations. Atypical orientations are interpretive standpoints for redefining the purposes of and possibilities available within institutional interactions.

For me, resolving the seeming contradiction that institutional discourses are both predictable and unpredictable directs attention to the artfulness of participants in institutional interactions. Participants display their interactive and interpretive skills in responding to the practical issues emergent in social interactions. They include issues that the institutions are designed to address and atypical developments. Different institutions provide participants with different resources in negotiating their relationships with each other and mutually agreeable responses to clients' concerns. Thus, we must attend to the details of institutional interactions in appreciating participants' artfulness in managing institutional interactions.

Consider, for example, the challenges faced by physicians in telling parents about their children's long-term developmental disabilities (Maynard, 1991) and family mediators in negotiating child custody agreements between angry divorcing spouses (Garcia, 1991). Physicians' and family mediators' options vary based on their general social standing in society (particularly as authorities on clients' problems), access to tests, procedures and documents that support their assessments, and the consequences of failing to reach agreements about the issues at hand. Maynard (1991) analyzes how physicians move interactions with parents toward medically prescribed resolutions, whereas family mediators' skills involve artfully managing potential disputes by encouraging spouses to find common ground about their future rights and responsibilities as parents (Garcia, 1991). Physicians' and family mediators' differing options point to power differences in professional-client interactions. Some professionals are better positioned to realize the traditional North American concept of professionalism than others.

Two challenges are particularly important for understanding discursive therapy interactions. The first is the availability of alternative discourses to clients in describing their concerns and assessing possible responses to them. Discursive therapy settings are not islands disconnected from the discourses of the larger society nor are all participants in the settings equally receptive to discursive therapy discourse. The second potential challenge involves the changing circumstances of clients' lives over the course of therapy relationships. The changes may give rise to new issues having potentially significant implications for subsequent therapist-client interactions, including changes that undercut therapists' and clients' prior working agreements about how to talk about clients' lives. Thus, negotiation is an ongoing activity shaping the possibilities for collaboration in therapist-client interactions. I discuss the relevance of ethnomethodology, conversation analysis, and Foucauldian discourse studies for understanding discursive therapy interactions as negotiations in the next section.

Studying Discursive Therapy Interactions

Ethnomethodology, conversation analysis, and Foucauldian discourse studies are strategies for conceptualizing and observing discursive therapist-client interactions. They highlight different aspects of how institutionally preferred realities are constructed and contested in the interactions. Ethnomethodological and conversation analyses focus on participants' practices within interactions, whereas Foucauldian scholars often explore the larger societal and historical contexts of institutional discourses. While their differences should not be minimized, these research strategies are similar to each other and the institutional discourse of discursive therapies in stressing how institutional realities are "ways of understanding and being in social worlds" (Miller, 1994, p. 282). They organize and justify forms of action.

Ethnomethodology

Ethnomethodologists analyze institutional realities as accounts that cast people's experiences as reflecting the facts of their lives (Garfinkel, 1967; Heritage, 1984; Pollner, 1987). Accounts construct social realities that people treat as existing separate from their interpretations of events and objects in their worlds. Accounts are standpoints for understanding what is going on in situations and what to expect as they unfold. This approach to institutional discourse is well suited to ethnographic research strategies because it focuses on how people use language in socially constructing the multiple contexts of their lives. Ethnomethodologists describe people's practical uses of accounts in advancing their interests in situations.

Consider Smith's (1978) study of how members of a student group socially constructed another member (K) as mentally ill by describing numerous concrete events that—by themselves—might be interpreted as unusual but not clear evidence of mental illness. She documents how social categories are cast as facts by linking observable events together to form patterns of meaning. Thus, the credibility of the students' account rested on how each description extended the mental illness claims of the other descriptions. The account justified group members' efforts to remove K from the group. Smith's (1978) study illustrates ethnomethodologists' emphasis on the interpretive practices that people use in constructing social realities.

Accounts are mutable social realities because they may be modified and even replaced by alternative social constructions within interactions. Alternative realities may emerge in response to changing circumstances that make persons' past ways of making sense inappropriate or as new storylines for organizing people's accounts of their lives. New storylines need not compel people to change; rather, they may be constructed as additional possibilities for orienting to situations. Raising new storylines is a fundamental activity in discursive therapist-client interactions. Discursive therapists raise them in a variety of ways, such as by asking about times when clients' problems are less severe and encouraging clients to externalize their problems (De Jong & Berg, 2002; White & Epston, 1990).

Ethnomethodologists also describe the complexities of facilitating change in clients' lives. The complexities include people's capacities for adapting their accepted accounts to explain their changed life circumstances. This brings us back to Smith's (1978) study of the methodical way in which students constructed K as mentally ill. Discursive therapists do not ask magical questions that stand alone in transforming their clients' lives. Rather, they use linked questions and comments to extend clients' accounts toward preferred storylines. Sutherland, Diehart, and Turner (2013) analyze such practices as therapeutic persistence. Discursive therapists persist by following up on client responses that they deem promising and ignoring those assessed as unpromising. These practices direct attention to the close connection between interpretation and interaction in discursive therapist-client negotiations. This connection is also central to the conversation analytic approach to discursive therapies.

Conversation Analysis

Conversation analysts closely examine audio and video recordings of institutional interactions. Their research considers participants' orientations to their own and others' institutional statuses, opportunities to participate, and rhetorical practices in their interactions. Conversation analysts' studies display the artful ways in which people sustain institutional realities while also pursuing their own interests in interactions by examining the procedures that organize social interactions. The procedures include multiple forms of turn-taking (who speaks and who listens when) and elicitations of responses from others (e.g., question-answer, call-response, description-elaboration sequences).

These procedures are related to the general social expectation that persons' responses to others' prior utterances will somehow fit with the prior utterances (Sacks, 1987). This is not to say that responses that violate the expectation are treated as irrelevant, rather, they are meaningful but in different ways than responses that fulfill social expectations. Think about how you respond to people who do not return your customary greetings (e.g., "Good morning") or conversation initiations (e.g., "How are you?"). Sacks (1992, p. 169) characterizes these procedures as a machine that "spews out" orderly social interactions. The procedures do not determine what is said; rather, they guide participants' actions in interacting with one another.

Conversation analysts' close examinations of social interactions provide data for documenting the concrete ways that people monitor one another's actions and use their turns at talk and listening to move their interactions in preferred directions. This is how language is a social activity for conversation analysts. The recordings display how new meanings emerge in the back and forth of interactions, and how participants mark some statements as more significant than others. For example, Martinez (2014) explains that one way that discursive therapists mark client statements as significant is by making their listening visible to clients, such as by repeating clients' words in therapists' subsequent questions or comments.

A major theme in conversation analytic studies of discursive therapists' interactional practices involves therapists' use of formulations (Georgaca & Advi, 2009; Korman, Bavelas, & DeJong, 2013; Muntigl & Horvath, 2014). Formulations are statements that reframe selected aspects of others' statements, making them fit with one's preferred versions of social reality (Garfinkel & Sacks, 1970). Discursive therapists often use formulations in responding to clients' depictions of their lives as ongoing struggles by treating the struggles as signs of clients' resilience, tenacity, or commitment to family. Formulations are central to discursive therapists' persistent encouragement of institutionally preferred storylines in interactions with clients.

Kurri and Wahlström (2005) have extended conversation analysis of formulations in discursive therapies in discussing how a team of therapists reframed a married couple's blaming of each other for their marital problems. The therapists' collectively and humorously built a formulation that cast the spouses as sharing the same desires about their relationship, even as they acted in ways that made their problems worse. The therapists further "softened" their preferred interpretation by describing hypothetical clients experiencing the same feelings as the actual clients. Kurri and Wahlström's study illustrates conversation analysts' interest in both what is said in interactions and how it is said.

Foucauldian Discourse Studies

Foucauldian discourse scholars conceptualize institutional discourses as historically variable constellations of rules and practices that shape what people can and cannot say in social interactions (Hall, 1997; Shumway, 1989). The rules and practices organize gazes, that is, culturally approved ways of perceiving and responding to issues in life. Foucault emphasizes how historical periods involve their own social realities that are sustained in distinctive gazes and institutional discourses. For example, Foucault (1973) traces the modern concept of disease as conditions arising within the body to the emergence of a new institutional discourse during the eighteenth century. This clinical gaze privileged physicians' medical knowledge and practices by rendering them as authoritative standpoints for comprehending the human body.

Foucauldian discourse scholars emphasize how social realities are constructed within power relations. While institutional discourses often privilege some participants' interests over others, Foucault (1977) adds that the concept of power relations includes the ways that all participants' contribute to the construction of institutionally approved social realities. We see this process in observing how socially honored orientations to body and health, crime and procedural fairness, and knowledge are affirmed by participants in medical examinations, courtroom procedures, and the testing of students in school.

For Foucauldian scholars, institutional discourses are conditions of possibility. They are organized to produce one or a few preferred social realities, although other realities may emerge within them. Dispreferred social realities are possible because all aspects of institutional discourses are not consistent, nor do the discourses operate fully independent from other social contexts (Foucault, 1972). Conditions of possibility are also shaped by the differing orientations to social reality available to participants in multi-discursive settings. For example, Moore and Seu (2010) have identified three discourses in clients' portrayals of their experiences in family therapy: medical, counseling, and consumerist discourses. The clients described the discourses as facilitating different therapy goals and definitions of clients' capacities for self-determination.

Ethnomethodologists and conversation analysts have taken up issues raised by Foucauldian discourse scholars in examining discursive therapist-client interactions. The studies represent one approach to clarifying social processes that organize power relations in discursive therapies. For example, Miller and Silverman (1995) describe how family therapy and solution-focused brief therapy interactions orient to a discourse of enablement that positions clients as free to choose how they wish to go on with their lives and therapists as skilled enablers of clients' decision-making. Hutchby (2007) extends this approach in considering how discursive child counselors invite clients to express "authentic" emotions, concerns, and hopes about their lives and selves. He shows how children are constructed as therapeutic subjects who are able to discuss such matters in institutionally preferred ways.

Miller and Silverman's (1995) and Hutchby's (2007) studies illustrate how therapists and clients are assigned institutionally preferred competencies and responsibilities within the conditions of possibility of discursive therapy discourse. The social construction of this preferred institutional reality may break down, however, when therapists or clients act in ways that significantly depart from typical interactional practices. For example, Hutchby describes how the children in his study interrupted typical counseling interactions by insisting that they could not answer the counselors' questions. The counselors' treated the children's actions as undermining the conditions necessary for counselor-child collaboration. I turn to collaboration in discursive therapies in the next section.

Collaboration in Discursive Therapies?

Ethnomethodological, conversation analytic, and Foucauldian discourse studies explore the processes through which institutionally preferred realities are constructed in institutional settings. I see these and related discursive perspectives in the social sciences as forming a paradigm, a body of assumptions and concerns that organize the inquiries of members of scientific communities (Kuhn, 1970). Paradigms are contexts for generating questions about aspects of the worlds in which we live. They are standpoints for reflection and discovery. Paradigms foster conversations about matters of shared concern within scientific and other communities. I develop this aspect of discursive social science in this section by discussing some ways that ethnomethodological, conversation analytic, and Foucauldian discourse research might cultivate conversations about discursive therapist-client collaboration.

Concern for collaboration is a pervasive theme in discursive therapists' depictions of their interactions with clients. Collaboration is a rubric within discursive therapy discourse. Discursive therapists use it in categorizing diverse approaches within the therapy world, as a summarizing term encompassing several related claims about how therapy should be practiced, and in justifying their practices to others. The claim is also fundamental to discursive therapists' reluctance to characterize their discourse as an institution. Consistent with their discourse, discursive therapists typically portray their interactions with clients as conversations.

While it is often framed as a moral choice, collaboration may also be interpreted as a practical accommodation to the conditions of discursive therapist-client interactions. So viewed, collaboration is a shared therapist-client work project. Analyzing such work is an important theme in ethnomethodological, conversation analytic, and Foucauldian discourse research. I discuss three directions for conversations about collaboration in discursive therapies in this section. They involve focusing on when and how collaboration happens, examining how collaborative relations are built and break down within therapist-client interactions, and analyzing discursive therapy interactions as sites of multi-discursive engagement.

From "What is it?" to "When and How is it?"

"What is it?" is a ubiquitous question in institutional discourses in Western cultures. It assumes that the issue at hand is sufficiently stable that it can be described and categorized. Consider, for example, the related claims to "not knowing" and "leading from one step behind" made by collaborative and solution-focused brief therapy therapists about their relationships with clients. Anderson (1997) defines not knowing as an attitude of continuing curiosity about clients' experiences and desires for their lives. She adds that this attitude is fundamental to collaborative therapists' efforts to work with—not on—their clients. De Jong and Berg (2002) echo this claim in stating that leading from one step behind is a way of recognizing that clients are experts on their own lives and how their lives might be changed.

The literature written by collaborative and solution-focused brief therapists treats not knowing and leading from one step behind as an enduring therapist attitude. Thus, one might look for evidence of it in assessing whether a particular therapy interaction is "truly" collaborative or solution-focused. Finding such evidence may, however, involve some complications. The complications turn on when and how therapists decide what client statements warrant a not knowing or leading from one step behind response and clients' responses to therapists' actions. These aspects of discursive interactions point to how the work of collaboration is an ongoing and shifting process of negotiation. What counts as collaboration at one point in a therapy interaction may not count at other points.

Consider, for example, the fine line that sometimes separates people's interpretations of others' questions as expressions of appropriate interest and unwarranted intrusions into their personal lives. Discursive therapists also risk being accused of inauthenticity if they continue to express curiosity about issues that clients have previously discussed and consider settled. To be fair, some discursive therapist writers—including Anderson (1997) and De Jong and Berg (2002)—have discussed how therapist-client collaboration evolves within and across therapy interactions, including suggesting questions that therapists might ask at different points in therapy relationships (Freedman & Combs, 1996).

Missing from this literature are descriptions of the collaborative competencies displayed by discursive therapists and clients in negotiating their therapy relationships. White and Stancombe (2003) analyze such collaborative processes as reflection in action. It consists of the seemingly intuitive ways that therapists and clients react as they listen to each other's words and observe their nonverbal actions. Reflection in action is the practical expertise that people use in managing shifting and sometimes unpredictable interactions. White and Stancombe stress the usefulness of ethnomethodological and conversation analytic studies in making reflection in action visible.

A potentially significant line of inquiry consists of explorations of collaborative therapist-client negotiations over the course of entire therapy sessions (Gale, 1991). This research focus orients to how therapists and clients continuously construct conditions for different forms of collaboration, disagreement, and disalignment, and to the methods they use in repairing interactions that therapists or clients assess as unsatisfactory. The studies might also analyze how discursive therapists and clients reconstruct prior forms of collaboration at later points in their interactions. Each of these possibilities for collaboration and disalignment in discursive therapy interactions may be further developed through the concept of power relations.

Power, Collaboration, and Entrapment in Therapist-Client Interactions

It is perhaps not surprising that discussion of power in discursive therapy interactions is largely absent from the conventional wisdom professed by discursive therapists. Indeed, this theme is seldom mentioned in the writings of discursive therapists who draw on Foucauldian perspectives in explaining how their clients are negatively affected by social practices associated with dominant institutional discourses in Western societies. This absence is unfortunate because, in failing to engage the issue, discursive therapists forego opportunities to expand upon Foucault's observations about how power is integral to productive processes in social interactions. Changes in clients' lives initiated in discursive therapy interactions are constituted in the exercise of power by therapists and clients (Sutherland & Strong, 2011).

Foucault states that power is observable in the ways that people use their positions in social interactions to influence one another (Bess, 1988). He characterizes power relations as unbalanced because different positions in social interactions provide access to different resources for influencing others. These resources involve both coercive tactics and diverse techniques of persuasion. Particularly relevant to therapists' power position are their institutional status as professional problem-solvers and the social expectation that therapists will ask questions that clients answer. These conditions facilitate discursive therapists' efforts to advance institutionally preferred social realities by persistently asking questions about clients' lives. Of course, clients do sometimes challenge the presuppositions of their therapists' questions and emotionally withdraw from the interactions (Muntigl & Horvath, 2014). They also use "yes, but" and subtler expressions in resisting their therapists' efforts to shape their interactions (Ekberg & LeCouteur, 2015; MacMartin, 2008; Muntigl, 2013).

Foucault cautions that the back and forth flow of influence between participants in interaction can break down and be replaced by coercive relations in which one or more participants impose their power on others (Bess, 1988). He portrays this development as the freezing of situations in ways that immobilize the participants; negotiation ceases and is replaced by demands for acquiescence. Foucault adds that frozen situations result from advantaged participants becoming trapped in their own discourses. They lose their sense of the multiple possible power relations that might be constructed within institutional discourses.

Nylund and Corsiglia (1994) depict frozen interactions as solution-forced rather than solution-focused. Discursive therapists subvert negotiation by persistently asking questions about matters that do not interest clients and demanding that clients pursue therapists' preferred goals (cf. Hutchby, 2007). For example, discursive therapists become trapped in their institutional discourse by insisting that clients describe times when their problems are less severe or absent, construct accounts that fit with therapists' assumptions about what counts as a useful life story and rejecting client claims to not knowing the answer to therapists' questions. These practices transform therapy interactions into scripts that position therapists and clients in restricted roles limiting their opportunities for multi-discursive engagement.

Discursive Therapy Discourse as Multi-discursive Engagement

Emerson and Messinger (1977) have examined how institutional responses to personal and social problems are associated with larger arrangements of power in society. Some institutions are given public license to impose institutionally preferred remedies on clients and the public, whereas other institutions have developed without such power. Emerson and Messinger (1977, p. 129) explain that professional-client relations in the latter institutions are typically symmetrical, that is, a professional "has to negotiate a mutually acceptable settlement relying upon personal resources and sanctions." This is the social context in which the discursive therapy discourses emerged as environments fostering collaboration.

It is perhaps obvious but still important to point out that the availability of alternative discourses is a necessary condition for the negotiation of mutually agreeable understandings in symmetrical professional-client relationships. Discursive therapy discourse cannot function without clients describing their lives in ways that depart from the institutional discourse of discursive therapies. Clients' use of alternative discourses might be characterized as the energy needed for discursive therapy discourse to operate. Recognition of this condition is fundamental to the attitude of not knowing and leading from one step behind. It is related to discursive therapists' use of formulations, scaling and optimistic questions, and attempts to externalize clients' problems. They are rhetorical devices designed to persuade—not compel—clients to interpret their lives in institutionally preferred ways.

Treating discursive therapy discourse as multi-discursive engagement highlights the importance of research on how and when discursive therapists and clients collaborate. Their interactions are transformative to the extent that therapists and clients construct resources for initiating change in clients' lives. The resources are socially constructed as therapists and clients bring together aspects of multiple discourses to produce new meanings that are, at least partly, unique to the interactions in which they were constructed. A multi-discursive perspective challenges the idea that discursive therapist-client interactions turn on clients being experts on their lives and therapists on eliciting therapeutically useful information from clients. Close examinations of therapist-client interactions show clients' expertise in helping their therapists ask useful questions and therapists' contributions to clients' storytelling (Miller, 2014).

A multi-discursive perspective on discursive therapy negotiations calls attention to how therapists and clients collaboratively reflect in action. It reminds us to pay attention to how therapists' decisions about what to say next are related to clients' prior questions or comments. Through multi-discursive negotiation, discursive therapists and clients guide each other toward mutually agreeable meanings that clients might treat as starting points for changing their lives. A multi-discursive perspective is also helpful in seeing how discursive therapists become trapped in their institutional discourse by ceasing engagement with alternative discourses. An important question that discursive therapists and researchers might address in their conversations asks, "How do therapists and clients remobilize themselves by re-engaging with multiple discourses available within their interactions?"

Conclusion

I have applied an institutional discourse perspective to discursive therapies in this paper. The perspective stresses the interconnections between the languages, assumptions, and practical interests organizing institutional settings. It is a framework for analyzing how institutionally preferred social realities are constructed in social interaction. I have drawn on aspects of ethnomethodology, conversation analysis, and Foucauldian discourse studies in discussing the social organization of discursive therapist-client collaboration. These research strategies are particularly helpful in seeing the multiple facets of collaboration in discursive therapies. Collaboration is a social value professed by discursive therapists, practical accommodation to symmetrical therapist-client relationships, shifting accomplishment that therapists and clients continuously work at in their interactions, organized within therapist-client power relations, and a context for socially constructing multi-discursive realities.

Each of these aspects of collaboration in discursive therapies might be further developed in future research. Other studies might examine related social values professed by discursive therapists, such as discursive therapists' portrayals of their own and clients' positions as experts in their interactions. I have also suggested that therapists' and clients' interactional contributions intersect in ways that are not recognized in the discursive therapy literature. Empirical studies of therapist-client contributions may extend our understanding of how helping or enabling relationships are organized in discursive therapy interactions.

Research on these issues has potential implications for discursive researchers' positioning of clients in their studies. The studies often involve therapist-centric assumptions about therapists' and clients' influence within their interactions. In particular, discursive researchers are inclined to emphasize therapists' actions in repairing potentially troubled therapy relationships while marginalizing how clients' "resistant" acts advance their interests in the interactions. Foregrounding clients' actions in power relations with therapists may also help researchers to see the many subtle ways that clients shape how they and their lives are socially constructed in discursive therapies, including introducing aspects of alternative discourses into accounts that appear to be only responsive to therapists' questions and comments.

Whatever its concrete focus, discursively oriented research on the institutional discourse of discursive therapies promises to reveal the complex processes operating in therapist-client interactions (Miller & McKergow, 2012). It may enrich discursive therapists' understandings of their professional values and appreciation of their clients' interactional competencies.

References

Anderson, H. (1997). *Conversation, language, and possibilities: A postmodern approach to therapy*. New York, NY: Basic Books.

Anderson, H., & Gehart, D. (Eds.). (2007). *Collaborative therapy: Relationships and conversations that make a difference* (pp. 7–20). New York, NY: Routledge.

Bess, M. (1988). Foucault interview: Power, moral values, and the intellectual. *History of the Present, 4*, 11–13.

De Jong, P., & Berg, I. K. (2002). *Interviewing for solutions* (2nd ed.). Pacific Grove, CA: Brooks/Cole Publishing Company.

Ekberg, K., & LeCouteur, A. (2015). Clients' resistance to therapists' proposals: Managing epistemic and deontic status. *Journal of Pragmatics, 90*, 12–25.

Emerson, R. M., & Messinger, S. L. (1977). The micro-politics of trouble. *Social Problems, 25*, 121–135.

Foucault, M. (1972). *The archaeology of knowledge* (A. M. S. Smith, Trans.). New York, NY: Harper & Row, Publishers.

Foucault, M. (1973). *The birth of the clinic: An archaeology of medical perception* (A. M. S. Smith, Trans.). New York, NY: Random House, Inc.

Foucault, M. (1977). *Discipline and punish: The birth of the prison* (A. Sheridan, Trans.). New York, NY: Random House, Inc.

Freedman, J., & Combs, G. (1996). *Narrative therapy: The social construction of preferred realities*. New York, NY: W. W. Norton & Company.

Gale, J. E. (1991). *Conversation analysis of therapeutic discourse*. Norwood, NJ: Ablex.

Garcia, A. (1991). Dispute resolution without disputing: How the interactional organization of mediation hearings minimizes argument. *American Sociological Review, 56*, 818–835.

Garfinkel, H. (1967). *Studies in ethnomethodology*. Englewood Cliffs, NJ: Prentice-Hall, Inc.

Garfinkel, H., & Sacks, H. (1970). On formal structures of practical actions. In J. C. McKinney & E. A. Tiryakian (Eds.), *Theoretical sociology: Perspectives and developments* (pp. 337–366). New York, NY: Appleton-Century-Crofts.

Georgaca, E., & Advi, E. (2009). Evaluating the talking cure: The contribution of narrative, discourse, and conversation analysis to psychotherapy assessment. *Qualitative Research in Psychology, 6*, 233–247.

Hacker, P. M. S. (2013). The linguistic turn in analytic philosophy. In M. Beaney (Ed.), *The Oxford handbook of the history of analytic philosophy* (pp. 926–947). Oxford: Oxford University Press.

Hall, S. (1997). The work of representation. In S. Hall (Ed.), *Representation: Cultural representations and signifying practices* (pp. 72–81). London: Sage.

Heritage, J. (1984). *Garfinkel and ethnomethodology*. Cambridge: Polity Press.

Holstein, J. A., & Gubrium, J. F. (Eds.). (2008). *Handbook of constructionist research*. New York, NY: The Guilford Press.

Hughes, E. C. (Ed.). (1971). *The sociological eye: Selected papers on work, self and the study of society*. Chicago, IL: Aldine Atherton.

Hutchby, I. (2007). *The discourse of child counselling*. Amsterdam: John Benjamins Publishing Company.

Korman, H., Bavelas, J. B., & DeJong, P. (2013). Microanalysis of formulations in solution-focused brief therapy, cognitive behavioral therapy, and motivational interviewing. *Journal of Systemic Therapies, 32*, 31–45.

Kuhn, T. S. (1970). *The structure of scientific revolutions*. Chicago, IL: University of Chicago Press.

Kurri, K., & Wahlström, J. (2005). Placement of responsibility and moral reasoning in couple therapy. *Journal of Family Therapy, 27*, 352–369.

Lock, A., & Strong, T. (2010). *Social constructionism: Sources and stirrings in theory and practice*. Cambridge: Cambridge University Press.

Lock, A., & Strong, T. (Eds.). (2012). *Discursive perspectives in the therapeutic practice*. Oxford: Oxford University Press.

MacMartin, C. (2008). Resisting optimistic questions in narrative and solution-focused therapies. In A. Peräylä, C. Antaki, S. Vehiläinen, & I. Leudar (Eds.), *Conversation analysis and psychotherapy* (pp. 80–99). Cambridge: Cambridge University Press.
Martinez, A. I. (2014). Collaborative forms of talk in supervision: A view from discursive psychology. *International Journal of Collaborative Practice, 5*, 98–116.
Maynard, D. W. (1991). The perspective-display series in the delivery and receipt of diagnostic news. In D. Boden & D. H. Zimmerman (Eds.), *Talk and social structure: Studies in ethnomethodology and conversation analysis* (pp. 164–194). Berkeley, CA: University of California Press.
Miller, G. (1994). Toward ethnographies of institutional discourse: Proposal and suggestions. *Journal of Contemporary Ethnography, 23*, 280–306.
Miller, G. (2014). Culture in solution-focused consultation: An intercultural approach. *Journal of Solution-Focused Brief Therapy, 1*, 25–40.
Miller, G., & McKergow, M. (2012). From Wittgenstein, complexity and narrative emergence: Discourse and solution-focused brief therapy. In A. Lock & T. Strong (Eds.), *Discursive perspectives in therapeutic practice* (pp. 163–183). New York, NY: Oxford University Press.
Miller, G., & Silverman, D. (1995). Troubles talk and counseling discourse: A comparative study. *The Sociological Quarterly, 36*, 725–747.
Moore, L., & Seu, I. B. (2010). 'Doing family therapy': A foucauldian discourse analysis. *European Journal of Psychotherapy & Counselling, 12*, 323–343.
Muntigl, P. (2013). Resistance in couples counselling: Sequences of talk that disrupt progressivity and promote disaffiliation. *Journal of Pragmatics, 49*, 18–37.
Muntigl, P., & Horvath, A. O. (2014). The therapeutic relationship in action: How therapists and clients co-manage relational disaffiliation. *Psychotherapy Research, 24*, 327–345.
Nylund, D., & Corsiglia, V. (1994). Being solution-focused forced in brief therapy: Remembering something important we already knew. *Journal of Systemic Therapies, 31*, 5–12.
Pollner, M. (1987). *Mundane reason: Reality in everyday life and sociological discourse*. Cambridge: Cambridge University Press.
Ray, W. A. (1999). Introduction: The relevance of brief therapy in the current managed care environment. In W. A. Ray & S. d. Shazer (Eds.), *Evolving brief therapies: In honor of John H. Weakland* (pp. xviii–xvxxv). Galena, IL: Geist & Russell Companies.

Sacks, H. (1987). On the preference for agreement and contiguity in sequences in conversation. In G. Button & J. R. E. Lee (Eds.), *Talk and social organisation* (pp. 54–69). Clevedon, Avon: Multilingual Matters.
Sacks, H. (1992). *Lectures on conversation: Volumes I & II*. Oxford: Blackwell.
Shumway, D. R. (1989). *Michel Foucault*. Charlottesville: University Press of Virginia.
Smith, D. E. (1978). 'K is mentally ill': The anatomy of a factual account. *Sociology, 12*, 23–53.
Strong, T., & Lock, A. (2005). Discursive therapy? *Janus Head, 8*, 585–593.
Sutherland, O., Diehart, A., & Turner, J. (2013). Responsive persistence part II. Practices of postmodern therapies. *Journal of Marital and Family Therapy, 39*, 488–501.
Sutherland, O., & Strong, T. (2011). Therapeutic collaboration: A conversation analysis of constructionist therapy. *Journal of Family Therapy, 33*, 256–278.
Tarragona, M. (2008). Postmodern/poststructuralist therapy. In J. L. Lebow (Ed.), *21st century psychotherapies* (pp. 167–205). Hoboken, NJ: John Wiley & Sons.
Weakland, J. H. (1999). That was then, this is now—Some further thoughts. In W. A. Ray & S. d. Shazer (Eds.), *Evolving brief therapies: In honor of John H. Weakland* (pp. 209–219). Galena, IL: Geist & Russell Companies.
Weinberg, D. (2008). The philosophical foundations of constructionist research. In J. A. Holstein & J. F. Gubrium (Eds.), *Handbook of constructionist research* (pp. 13–40). New York, NY: Guilford Press.
White, M. (2007). *Maps of narrative practice*. New York, NY: W. W. Norton & Company.
White, M., & Epston, D. (1990). *Narrative means to therapeutic ends*. New York, NY: W. W. Norton & Company.
White, S., & Stancombe, J. (2003). *Clinical judgement in the health and welfare professions: Extending the evidence base*. Philadelphia: Open University Press.

6

Reflexive Questions as Constructive Interventions: A Discursive Perspective

Joaquín Gaete, Olga Smoliak, and Shari Couture

This chapter aims to promote dialogue between discursive-oriented researchers (e.g., Potter & Hepburn, 2007) and therapists (e.g., Lock & Strong, 2012). Both share an interest in therapy talk as "reflexive": they approach discourse as a form of joint action rather than as information that goes through a tube (e.g., Edwards, 1997; Tomm, 1988). At the same time, they clearly differ in aims and "methods" of inquiry. Discursive therapists seem to be interested in optimizing therapy and, therefore, deliberately using reflexivity in client-responsive ways. They do it by theorizing about therapy practice using (theory-charged) concepts such as

J. Gaete (✉)
Universidad Adolfo Ibáñez, Viña del Mar, Chile
e-mail: joaquin.gaete@uai.cl

O. Smoliak
Department of Family Relations and Applied Nutrition, University of Guelph, Guelph, ON, Canada
e-mail: osmoliak@uoguelph.ca

S. Couture
Calgary, AB, Canada

O. Smoliak, T. Strong (eds.), *Therapy as Discourse*, The Language of Mental Health,
https://doi.org/10.1007/978-3-319-93067-1_6

"clients' preferences." They may talk of "absent but implicit" values (White, 2003); "preferred" identities and other developments in clients' lives (e.g., Freedman & Combs, 1996); collaborative or subject-subject type of therapeutic relationships (e.g., Weingarten, 1992); and clients' autonomy (Tomm, 1988). On the other hand, discursive-oriented researchers are less concerned with abstract concepts depicting therapy talk and its "outcomes" and more with how participants in a specific interaction use language, in observable ways, and for what local social purposes.

In this chapter, we explore how drawing on both discursive (therapeutic and research) perspectives may help deepen understanding and enrich practice of discursive therapy. Our focus is on a specific discursive therapy practice—reflexive questions (Tomm, 1987b, 1988). Reflexive questions can be used to constitute "preferred" descriptions and understandings of clients' relationships, identities, and actions. Drawing from discursive researchers, specifically discursive psychologists, we suggest that reflexive questions invite conversational "attribution work." Discursive psychologists approach *attributions* as talk-in-action rather than as individual cognitive processes. In particular, they investigate how psychological matters (e.g., emotions, cognitions, identities) are formulated, ascribed, and resisted by people engaged in social interaction (te Molder, 2015). Re-conceptualized in discursive terms, this attributting to people of traits, motives, affective states, resposibility, etc. (i.e., "attribution work") becomes empirically accessible to discursive therapists interested in co-constructing clients' identity and experience in client-responsive ways. In other words, a discursive-oriented lens on reflexive questions may enhance therapists' capacity to learn from and teach therapy practice: to learn, because it helps understand how discursive therapists use reflexivity therapeutically by asking reflexive questions and subsequently responding to clients' answers to accomplish clients' preferred versions of their experiences. To teach, as these investigations may help offer some ideas about how to make the use of such discursive reflexivity a more deliberate practice.

Enacting discursive reflexivity by asking reflexive questions invites a heightened ability to notice and orient to how the co-construction of alternative (deemed as preferred or helpful) meanings gets done, allowing therapists to participate in the therapeutic endeavor both responsively and collaboratively. Our main suggestion is that reflexive questions invite preferred attribution work. First we will elaborate on this theoretically, by unpacking the notion of reflexivity within both discursive practice and discursive research traditions. Then we will analyze segments of therapy talk to explore empirically the same idea.

Therapeutic Perspective on Reflexivity and Reflexive Questions

For therapists, everything they do in relation to clients is typically seen as a form of communication. Therapists cannot help but behave; therefore, they cannot help but communicate. This is, as Watzlawick, Beavin, and Jackson (1967) put it half a century ago, an "axiom" not just for therapy interaction, but for all human communication. As therapists, we may either consider seriously or ignore this axiom but, arguably, our stance will affect how the therapeutic conversation unfolds. This idea aligns with Karl Tomm's (1987a, 1987b, 1988) notion of "reflexivity" in his *interventive interviewing* framework for therapy and the first quote at the beginning of this chapter. Tomm proposed that "everything an interviewer does and says, and does not do and does not say is … an intervention that could be therapeutic, nontherapeutic, or countertherapeutic" (Tomm, 1987a, p. 4). For Tomm, even questions intended as mere information-gathering tools *are* interventions and will influence how the conversation unfolds, including the topics, activities, and presuppositions pursued and advanced in therapy. Regardless of intentions, every question a therapist offers favors and subtly advances particular understandings (e.g., ideas, actions, ways of being and relating). As a result, only certain topics, issues, or concerns get talked into being, and not others. We see meanings or understandings not as lifted from one person's mind and transferred to another person's mind but as jointly and interactionally worked up. As we discussed elsewhere (Sutherland, Sametband, Gaete, Couture, & Strong, 2013), such understandings are discursively accomplished as people produce, coordinate, and negotiate meaning through their interactions (see also, e.g., Berger & Luckmann, 1991; Shotter, 2008).

Tomm (1987b) suggested that therapists who seek to bring forth alternative possibilities for understanding and action may find reflexive questions useful. He defined reflexive questions as:

> Questions asked with the intent to facilitate self-healing in an individual or family by activating the reflexivity among meanings within preexisting belief systems that enable family members to generate or generalize constructive patterns of cognition and behavior on their own. (p. 4)

Some examples of reflexive questions include: "What are you worried might happen when your daughter stays out late?... What is the worst thing that comes to mind?" or "If you did raise these worries with her, do you think she would take it as a lack of trust? ... As an intrusion into her privacy? ... Or as an indication of your caring as a parent?" (Tomm, 1987b, p. 5). Reflexive questions may invite the construction of potentially useful understandings and courses of action previously not considered (e.g., parents disclosing their worries to the daughter rather than being critical of her behaviors). They can be used therapeutically to both modify (unhelpful or problematic) and/or stabilize (preferred) understandings, which in turn may modify/stabilize the practices and relationships sustained by such understandings (Tomm, 1987b).

Reflexive questions may help clients change their views and everyday practices and relationships (Tomm, 1987b). Linguistic distinctions embedded in questions and taken up in answers are, in this sense, political. As co-created, mutually acceptable conversational realities, they have power over those who generate and accept them as apt to understand or act within their world (see also Strong, 2007). Eventually, most therapists hope that clients will engage with these powerful distinctions (e.g., endorse, live by, apply) beyond the therapy room: this is how the constructive discursive process of therapy is typically expected to be influential in clients' extratherapeutic lives (Dreier, 2015), and this is how we interpret Tomm's idea of reflexive questions as facilitating "self-healing." For Tomm (1987a, 1987b), then, the associated therapeutic "effects" in these questions lies in two complementary sources of reflexivity, namely, (a) in how therapists' talk inevitably shapes clients' responses (and vice versa) and (b) in the shifting in meaning these questions trigger within clients' "belief systems."

Two Therapeutic Effects: Preferred Descriptions and Clients' Autonomy

With respect to the effects of reflexive questions, Tomm (1988) argued that both therapists and clients are likely to experience these questions as generative. Reflexive questions can help open space for new possibilities and help generate meanings/accounts that are deemed preferred (e.g., helpful, fitting, important) than previously held views (Tomm, 1988). These "preferred" realities include preferred descriptions of identities, practices, relationships, values, or emotions (e.g., Andersen, 1987; Combs & Freedman, 2012; Freedman & Combs, 1996; White, 2007; White & Epston, 1990). Accordingly, reflexive questioning can be seen as discursively accomplishing "preference work" in the sense that they help craft and invite continued co-construction of distinctions and meanings regarded as more preferable or helpful, as compared to prior meanings (Sutherland et al., 2013).

Reflexive questions may also have an effect of fostering client autonomy (Tomm, 1988). Proponents of various approaches to therapy increasingly strive to promote clients' participation, active engagement, self-exploration, and agency or capacity to self-heal or generate change on their own (see Bohart & Tallman, 2010; Gendlin, 1996; Gonzalez, 2016; Greenberg & Pinsoff, 1986; Orlinsky, Ronnestad, & Willutzki, 2004; Prochaska, DiClemente, & Norcross, 1992). Similarly, but invoking different reasons, discursive therapists have depicted therapy as a collaborative activity, respectful of clients' knowledge and agency, something that is done *with* rather than *to* clients (e.g., De Jong & Berg, 2002; Paré, 2012; Weingarten, 1992). Be it for pragmatic, ideological, or ethical reasons, there seems to be a growing consensus concerning the importance of relating to clients as subjects/agents (rather than objects/patients)

(Buber, 1970; Gadamer, 2004) and treating clients as individuals whose "lay" accounts on therapy and experience are comparable in legitimacy to professional explanations. Arguably, reflexive questions can be used to invite this type of subject-subject relationship between clients and therapists, wherein clients' knowledge is invited and treated as relevant and consequential and clients are seen as agents and active contributors of ideas rather than passive recipients of expert knowledge.

Tomm (1987b) suggested that therapists cannot determine clients' responses, because clients inevitably respond out of their own discursive capacities and background of meanings. Later Tomm (1988) contended that reflexive questioning invites clients to "make pertinent discoveries on their own" (p. 2). As a consequence, therapists may become not just more influential or effective, but more collaborative and ethical or, as Tomm (1988) put it, "their influencing intent is moderated by respect for the autonomy of clients" (p. 8). Tomm thus portrayed therapists' reflexive questions as deliberatively facilitative, enabling, or triggering rather than instructive, linear, or causally deterministic of clients' responses. The conceptual picture of reflexive questions clearly sets the stage for subject-subject therapeutic relationships and interactions to flourish.

To summarize, "reflexivity" in Tomm's therapeutic conception of reflexive questions could be described as having two key effects (which purportedly optimize the therapy process): they help generate alternative (preferred) understandings and they enable client autonomy or self-exploration. Let us now examine these effects from a discursive psychological research perspective. We will argue and demonstrate that discursive psychology can help bring to light features of therapy discourse and questioning practices that may be therapeutically relevant.

Discursive Psychological Perspective on Reflexive Questions and Their Effects

Discursive psychology (DP) (Edwards, 1997; Edwards & Potter, 1992; Hepburn & Wiggins, 2005; Potter, 2010; Tileagă & Stokoe, 2016; Wiggins, 2017) is an approach to the study of psychological phenomena (e.g., attribution, emotion, agency) from the perspective of participants in social interaction. DP scholars also see language use as "reflexive": not as transmitting information about people's mental life or the world but as a tool to accomplish social action. Claims of uncertainty ("I don't know"), for example, could be used in certain contexts to play down one's stake in a specific description (Potter, 1996). Complaints can be done in ways that manage inferences about the complainer (Edwards, 2005).

Drawing from DP, we approach the study of reflexive questions as interactional accomplishments. Descriptions are designed with the audience "in mind" or to be acceptable by their recipients. Discursive researchers can help understand how, specifically, affiliate with certain descriptions and how certain descriptions or "versions" of reality are locally established as more or less (mutually) acceptable. They can shed light on the rhetoric involved in issuing and responding to accounts offered in therapy, envisioning preferred or more acceptable meanings as a practical matter and discursive achievement of therapists and clients. From this perspective, the attention shifts away from preference as a matter that is internally formed (cognitive) and then outwardly expressed to preference as an interactional accomplishment.[1]

For the purposes of this chapter, we focus on attribution. Attribution is a form of describing concerned with how people make causal explanations of actions and events. Participants may invoke intents, interests, and motives or other explanatory devices of action as resources to accomplish social activities, such as blaming, inviting, or defending (Edwards & Potter, 1992). Attributional explanations do not have to be uttered directly (e.g., "he is to blame for our marital problems") and can be accomplished implicitly, for example, implied through factual descriptions of actions and events (e.g., "he's been working 24/7"). Speakers can attribute or ascribe certain traits or characteristics, sometimes in subtle or

[1] Discursive researchers have studied "preference" emphasizing how people construct their talk as more or less preferred (see Pomerantz & Heritage, 2013). For example, how speakers select certain ways of talking with particular interlocutors ("recipient design") or how certain kinds of initiating actions (invitations) normatively prefer or "expect" particular kinds of responses (acceptance). Notably conversation analysts relate preference to *affiliation*, or responses that endorse the teller's point of view (Lindström & Sorjonen, 2013). Since we focus on attribution, affiliation is the interactional phenomenon closest to our interest—generation of preferred meaning.

implicit ways, to themselves or others (te Molder, 2015). Issues of blame and accountability can be highly relevant in therapy, particularly in couple and family therapy where family members may have different perspectives on who is responsible for the "problem" and who needs to change (e.g., O'Reilly, 2014; Patrika & Tseliou, 2016; Stancombe & White, 2005). Applying a DP perspective to reflexive questions, such questions may be seen as ways to accomplish important attribution work—ascribe certain attributes to people or attribute causal sources of actions and events to certain sources (e.g., external or internal, situational or personal, temporal or permanent) in an effort to perform therapy-relevant social actions (e.g., blaming, justifying, excusing, requesting, complementing). We will suggest discursive-oriented therapists often see this type of work as co-constructing "preferred meanings" of their clients' life circumstances and identity (Tomm, 1987b, p. 4).

Let us revisit Tomm's (1987b) therapeutic conception of reflexive questions in an effort to recast it discursively. Tomm defined reflexive questions as:

> Questions asked with the intent to facilitate self-healing in an individual or family by activating the reflexivity among meanings within preexisting belief systems that enable family members to generate or generalize constructive patterns of cognition and behavior on their own. (p. 4)

DP scholars may argue that there are several features in this definition, such as the therapist's "intent" or clients' "self-healing" or "preexisting belief systems," that might be inconsistent with a DP perspective focused on social interaction rather than individual cognitive processes. As aforementioned, we see reflexive questions as opening space for co-construction and negotiation of "new" and mutually acceptable/preferred meanings and descriptions. Thus, the "reflexivity" of reflexive questions is not intrinsic to these questions, as suggested by Tomm (1987b), but is interactionally achieved. If we look back to our initial quotes, this conceptualization falls more in line with the second quote where reflexivity is accomplished as therapists become more responsively involved in the back and forth invited by these questions. Reflexive questions, as we will show, may embed "optimistic" presuppositions (MacMartin, 2008) or views of clients as positive people—resourceful, competent, and agentic. In their responses to reflexive questions, clients may take up (endorse, unpack, extend, etc.) such presuppositions. Accordingly, we would like to reformulate reflexive questioning in discursive terms as *questions that elicit, clarify, and unpack clients' reasoning—their explanations of and reflections on their own experiences.* As aforementioned, reflexive questions can (a) make available and ascribe to clients (through referring, hinting, evoking, etc.) certain psychological characteristics, or (b) explain clients' experiences and actions in particular ways (e.g., as caused by internal or external factors)—attributions which can then be take up or resisted by clients in their responses to questions.

We contend that our discursive-oriented reformulation helps make reflexive questions' constructive potential open to view, "since everything lies open to view there is nothing to explain" (Wittgenstein, 1953, p. 126). The "hidden" magic of the meaning-making process gets observable and understandable and, hence, teachable and learnable. Rather than speculating upon therapists' intent, as discursive researchers, we prefer to look for what observably happens in interaction as a consequence of therapists asking certain questions. We are interested in what happens after questions are posed, including how clients take up (or not) therapists' presuppositions and how therapists respond to clients' "resistant" responses to questions (de Shazer, 1984) observable, for instance, in clients' non-answers (e.g., MacMartin, 2008). From a micro-discursive perspective, we should be able to observe how clients and therapists mutually orient to the relevance of interactionally "centering" clients' reflections and explanations. Moreover, we should be able to see how alternative understandings of clients' experiences and identities—theorized effects of reflexive questions—are generated through social interaction.

Analyzing the Effects of Reflexive Questions

The exemplars below illustrate how reflexive questions can be examined discursively to better appreciate how discursive therapists and clients manage their responses to each other to stay in an intended zone of mutual preference. Exemplar 1a was taken from a family therapy process with Antonia, José, and their two children, Alex (17) and Sofía (12).[2] Exemplar 1a comes from a session with the parents alone. They had previously stated they wanted to address "violence issues" between them, to better address disruptive behaviors in their children, which was the original complaint. Prior to Exemplar 1a, the therapist (T) and José (J) had been talking about his "violent behavior." J shared an account for his violent behavior toward Antonia (A), stating that A usually insults him when she drinks too much alcohol, and that her alcohol consumption makes him "angry," makes him "lose control," and that he "reacts" with violence toward A. In line 114, T starts a sequence of reflexive questions about J's reaction. What makes these questions reflexive is that they elicit further explanations and reflections from the client. We can also observe how alternative (positive or non-pathologizing) distinctions or constructions of the client as a person and partner are produced through question-answer sequences of actions. In particular, we can see how T and J attribute certain attitudes and predispositions to J. Reflexive questions are highlighted (bolded) in each exemplar.

Exemplar 1a

114	T	**did you ever try to do something to not have the reaction you have**
115		**when Antonia drinks?**
116	J	yes
117	T	**what did you try?**
118	J	stop the fight and go away

In lines 114–115 and 117, T issues reflexive questions that elicit information from J concerning his prior attempts to react non-violently toward A. T's questions in lines 114–115 and in 117 are presupposi-

[2] These are English translations of data from a research project funded by the Government of Chile, Fondecyt project No. 11150198, approved by Universidad Adolfo Ibáñez' local Board of Ethics. Names are pseudonyms. Project involves the study of family therapy involving children with "disruptive behaviors." Data for this chapter were simplified to better suit its aims.

tional, that is, they tacitly advance certain assumptions about J's actions or attribute certain motives or intentions to J, namely that on rare occasions ("did you ever") he may have been doing something to prevent his violent reactions. In seeking, with a yes/no question (Raymond, 2003), J's confirmation that he has made attempts to abstain from violence (lines 114–115), T implicitly proposes that J's violent reactions are inappropriate or problematic (consider that any direct answer to a question treats the question's presuppositions as valid; Hayano, 2013; MacMartin, 2008). The use of vague or neutral language ("reaction"), as opposed to more specific, morally charged terms (e.g., "violence" or "abuse"), may be a way for T to attribute responsibility to J without being heard as critical or judgmental.

J's reactions are constituted as temporary and event-driven ("when Antonia drinks") rather than dispositional (e.g., J being an angry or violent person) (Edwards, 1999), which may be a way to present the "problem" as changeable and amenable to a therapeutic intervention. J's "reactions" are also presented as controllable or preventable (Edwards, 1999). J is distinguished not as a passive, non-agentic man who can do little about his reactions, but as a someone who has tried reacting non-violently. Once J confirms that he has attempted to act non-violently, T's information-seeking wh- (what) question (line 117) elicits details about J's prior attempts. In response, J endorses and exemplifies the proposed construction of him as an agentic subject—someone who has made efforts to act non-violently.

We can see how T and J orient to issues of blame and responsibility. This is evident in T advancing the notion that J is responsible for violence or that violence is morally problematic without sounding critical or judgmental, or in J joining the construction of himself as actively seeking to change his behavior. Responsibility and agency are attributed to J, that is, he is implicitly presented as responsible for his reactions and as actively attempting to act non-violently. J endorses the attribution of the motive to treat his partner in more caring, non-violent ways by supplying evidence of his attempts. Let us explore, in Exemplar 1b, how this interaction unfolds. Here, we see how an alternative description of the client's identity is offered (and endorsed) using a reflexive question.

Exemplar 1b

119	T	and how did Antonia respond?
120	J	she follows me
121	T	she follows you?
122	J	((nods))
123	T	**so what happens to you, what happens that makes you want to leave,**
124		**what is it that happens when you want to leave?**
125	J	so that I don't hit her
126	T	**that seems important to you not hitting her?**
127	J	yes ((nods))
128	T	**why is it important, José?**
129	J	because I think I still love her

T issues reflexive questions that elicit explanations (*why… because…; line 128*) and information from J concerning his intentions and values (line 123–124 and 126). J is mutually treated as more knowledgeable than T (Heritage, 2013) concerning J's mental life (motives, values, attitudes, etc.); it is *his* reflections and explanations that are sought and unpacked in this exchange. T's first question (line 124) recycles the information previously supplied by J ("stop the fight and go away," line 118). J is treated as more knowledgeable as compared to T about what promoted him to leave. T's question is reformulated mid-turn (lines 123–124) from "what happens that *makes* you want to leave" to "what is it that happens when you *want* to leave," which may be a way to constitute J as an agent with positive intentions, rather than a passive victim of his circumstances. T's question is formulated as variably interpretable: as eliciting information concerning, among others, Antonia's actions, other contextual factors, or J's emotional or mental states (e.g., feelings, intentions, thoughts, wishes, needs, etc.). Analytically, T's "actual" intentions in asking the question are irrelevant, as our analysis focuses on interactionally displayed interpretations of conduct—how T's question is "heard" or interpreted by J, which is observable in how J responds to the question. Line 125 shows that J hears T's question as being about *inten-*

tions behind J's "wanting to leave" ("so that I don't hit her"): J's leaving is constituted as an outcome of his (caring) intent to not hit A.

T's next declaratively formulated yes/no question (line 126) seeks confirmation from J of T's proposition that the intent to "not hit" is of significance to J, making available the inference concerning J being a certain kind of person (someone who is kind and concerned about his partner), the construction confirmed by J in the next turn (line 127). That is, the question implicitly assigns positive attributes to J. The question is mitigated with "seems" to downgrade T's knowledge of J's inner experience, namely, his values.

In lines 114–129 T issues a series of five reflexive questions. After accomplishing a description for a past event where J tried to behave differently ("stop the fight and go away"), T's questions invite J to account for this "exception," which they do by making relevant his "inner experience" or "values": both T and J accept this version where he *tried*, where he "*wanted* to leave," because he had "motive" ("so that I don't hit her"). T's last question (line 128) displays acceptance of J's ongoing version by inviting further accounting work (T elicits an explanation from J of the importance of not hitting A). J cites his continued (*still*) love for A as the reason, downgrading the certainty of his claim with *I think*. Issuing a non-committal or uncertain claim of love presents J as someone who has just realized that his efforts to not be violent might be motivated by his love for A. If he claimed his love for A more confidently, he may be accused of acting inconsistently with his claimed feelings for A. J's responses to T's questions help extend the construction of himself as a good person and partner and, perhaps, block the need to defend himself against the accusation that he is a violent person and "bad" partner. J's responses in lines 127 and 129 mark his affiliation with or endorsement ("yes," nod, unpacking with "because...") of T's claim that being non-violent carries importance for J. Here again, the therapist and the client co-construct (and implicitly accept, validate) an alternative account of J's identity through the use of reflexive questions.

We use Exemplar 1c to focus on the last two turns of Exemplar 1b (lines 128–129) in order to illustrate how reflexive questions may elicit "emotionally charged" accounts, which may in turn accomplish important attributional work (e.g., attribute certain attitudes or predispositions). This may be discursively "done" through very subtle features of talk, such as recognizable displays of upset. We use a more detailed transcription system here to include paraverbal and non-verbal aspects of talk (see the footnote for transcription notation).

Exemplar 1c[3]

128	T	**why is it important, José? [(10)**]
129	J	[(smiles, deeply inhales and exhales)]
130		because I think I still love her = (wobbly voice, aspiring, sniffing[4])
131	T	=Mh hm (6) how important (nods).
132	J	(nods) (3)
133	T	°Mmh° (3)

After T's question in line 128, we witness an enormous gap in the dialogue of ten seconds. In response, J performs several features of crying: whispering (note the ° ° sign), wobbly delivery, sniffing, deep breaths (Hepburn & Potter, 2012). T exhibits interest in J telling more with pauses and acknowledgment tokens (lines 131 and 133) (Jefferson, 1984). This "interested" response seems to validate (accept) J's performed, "emotive" explanation in line 130. T seems to recognize or "hear" (and accept) J's performance of "true pain," so to speak, the pain one feels when realizing and publicly acknowledging that one has hit and hurt his beloved. Displays of upset make certain inferences available about what kind of a person J is—someone who sincerely repents and cares. The dialogue continued with additional reflexive questioning (see Exemplar 1d).

[3] Numbers in parenthesis indicate time in seconds. Square parenthesis [ ] indicates an overlap of talk between J and T. Parenthesis ( ) indicates non-verbals. Talk between ° ° is quieter than surrounding talk (e.g., whispering). The sign "=" marks no discernible pause between the end of a speaker's utterance and the start of the next utterance.

[4] Hepburn and Potter (2012) characterize tremulous or wobbly delivery and aspiration as "a feature of speakers' attempts to talk through a crying episode" (p. 198), which seemed to be the case here. Sniffs were audible, defined as "inhalation, with the addition of various voiced vowels and consonants, caused by nasal or 'wet' sounds" (pp. 197–198).

Exemplar 1d

134	T	**and if there was a change José that you would like to do,**
135		**a minimal change, that you would like in your relationship with**
136		**Antonia, what would it be?**
137	J	that I would have to do?
138	T	you in your relationship with Antonia
139	J	to control myself more
140	T	**control myself in which sense?**
141	J	like this quick exploding, like yelling right away, swearing
142	T	**is this something important to you, José, being able to change that?**
143	J	yes, because maybe this way we can keep going

Exemplar 1d contains three reflexive questions. The first wh-question seeks information from J about relational changes he "would like to do." The second question elicits clarification of the meaning for J of "self-control." The last declaratively formulated with a rising intonation question seeks confirmation from J that enhancing self-control is important to J. Let us look more closely at these question-answer sequences.

In lines 134–136, T issues a hypothetical question (Peräkylä, 1995; Speer, 2012). The question describes a scenario in which J wishes to make changes in how he relates to A. The wh-question ("what would it be like," line 134) asks J to specify changes he "would like" to make. An extreme case formulation (Pomerantz, 1986) ("a *minimal* change") may be used to present T's proposal that J changes as reasonable and not excessive. J is implicitly asked to assume a small portion of responsibility for the couples' marital distress, rather than the entire responsibility. This may be done to undermine potential accusations of T being partial and unfair (siding with one partner against the other) and to enhance the likelihood that J endorses the idea of changing himself. Line 139 is hearable as J's eventual answer to T's hypothetical question ("to control myself more"), in which he endorses the attribution of responsibility for change to him. "More" is added to possibly imply that J has already exercised some degree of control over his actions.

With the second question T elicits clarification from J of the meaning of self-control ("control myself in which sense?"). With a three-part list ("quick exploding, yelling right away, swearing") (Jefferson, 1991) he exemplifies what he would not be doing if he had more self-control. T's use of an indexical ("this") in the next question treats the previous description as sufficiently clear/acceptable for the issue at hand. This last interrogatively formatted question (*is this …?*) seeking a *yes* response helps further center the discussion on the topic of J's changing himself and establish the relevance of self-change *for* J. The idea that J should change (i.e., enhance his self-control) is implicitly presented as stemming from J rather than as coming from T's agenda. J is discursively constructed as an agent and source of self-growth and self-improvement—as someone who is motivated to change, who cares, and who responds out of what is "important" to him. On line 143, J endorses ("yes") the notion that enhanced self-control is important to him and accounts for his agreement ("because…"). He attributes responsibility to himself for maintaining the relationship and implicitly assigns to himself the concern for his marriage and the attitude of caring for A. On line 143 we again see evidence of J affiliating with T's claim that self-change is important to J ("yes" and elaborating or unpacking "because…").

In the last exemplar below, the construction of J as a caring father, someone who seeks to instill certain values in his daughter, is "thickened" conversationally. Sara (11-year-old daughter) reacts by crying when she witnesses her parents fighting and asks J to not yell, which worries J.

Exemplar 1e

190	T	**why do you worry José when Sara tells you that?**
191	J	because I don't want her to think that
192		it is okay that they talk to you this way
193	T	so you don't want her to learn
194	J	the same pattern
195	T	**and instead of that José what is important to you that Sara learns?**
196	J	it is about being respected, that nobody can disrespect her

197 T it seems that that's important
198 J yes

The reflexivity of reflexive questions in lines 190 and 195 lies in the subsequent attributional work they observably elicit. The wh-question (line 190) elicits an account or explanation ("why… because…") from J of his emotional state ("worry") in response to his daughter's request that J does not yell at her mother. J provides such explanation in the next turn (lines 191–192). "They" in J's response presumably references either people in general or men. In the next turn (line 193), T formulates or summarizes ("so…") J's explanation, subtly reshaping its content from Sara *thinking* to Sara *learning*, highlighting J's fatherly role of a teacher and role model. Once again, J is attributed certain parenting attitudes and intentions; he is constituted as a father motivated by care and concern for his daughter. J completes T's utterance (line 194), which can be seen as a sign of his affiliation with or endorsement of T's claim that J "wants" to be a positive model to his daughter.

T's subsequent wh-question (line 195) builds on the material that has been previously established ("and instead of that") and elicits further information from J regarding the specifics of what J wants his daughter to learn from observing him, provided by J in the next turn. T's question once again attributes care to J and highlights the relevance and significance of positive fatherly intentions *for* him. J joints this construction by supplying information about values he seeks to instill in Sara (line 196). And once again, T's final turn (line 197) marks his limited access to J's mind by downgrading his statement with "seems." That is, T advances his ideas about J's experience while honoring J's superior knowledge of his own experience.

Both question-answer sequences work to attribute causality, presenting J's emotions and actions as stemming from his underlying positive fatherly intentions to teach his daughter good values. J may be accused of being a bad father who exposes his daughter to violence. We would argue that attributional work is done in service of defending against potential accusations that J exposes his own child to domestic violence. Indeed, we see that while T's first question more broadly elicits from J an explanation of his emotional state, J attributes positive intentions to himself in his response, arguably as a way to defend against potential accusations and attributions of blame. This highlights the importance of examining causal attributions while attending to the broader interactional context and social activities (e.g., defending, blaming, praising, complaining) oriented to and managed in interaction.

Discussion

In this chapter, we hoped to encourage a dialogue between discursive-oriented researchers and therapists. Our focus was on reflexive questions as constructive interventions. We offered a discursive psychological perspective on reflexive questions to better understand their potential effects for the therapeutic process: they invite attributional work. In doing so, they (a) help constructing mutually acceptable accounts; and (b) they foster the discursive construction of clients' autonomy (or capacity to generate preferred "patterns of cognition and behavior on their own"; Tomm, 1987b, p. 4).

In the exemplars we presented, T's questions opened space for the co-construction of alternative meanings and depictions of the client's actions and identity, namely, the construction of a morally acceptable (non-violent, kind, caring) partner and father identity. We have shown that questions were used to manage issues of blame and responsibility for change and accomplish attributional work—attribute agency, responsibility, and certain attitudes to the client. The client's actions were presented as causally linked or driven by his underlying values and intentions. The questions embedded and subtly advanced optimistic presuppositions about the client being a person motivated by "good" intentions and values (MacMartin, 2008). The client's positive intentions were topicalized (Vehviläinen, 2008) or presented as a relevant topic to explore in therapy and constituted as significant *for* the client. The client consistently endorsed the therapist's propositions concerning him being an agentic person, and the therapist systematically backed this up. Interestingly, the therapist treated the client as more knowledgeable than her in the accounting business (i.e., granting higher epistemic rights about clients' "inner" experience; Heritage, 2013), which some discursive-oriented *therapists* have long described as the enactment of a "not-knowing stance" (Anderson, 1997).

Tomm (1987b) offered a rich taxonomy of reflexive questions. What seems missing from his description is the back-and-forth conversational work involved in co-constructing alternative, client-preferred meanings. Rather than solely fixing our attention on carefully crafted questions, as therapists, we are able to orient to how alternative meanings is a collaborative endeavor: they are discursively generated in ongoing interaction. We highlighted that the micro-details of language use are not only relevant for therapists to pay attention to but are also consequential for how a conversation unfolds and which versions of clients' identities and experiences are advanced and constituted and which other possible versions are passed over. This perspective directs therapists' attention to the social interaction and discursive production of meaning in therapy (Avdi, 2005; Strong, 2007). As suggested in our second initial quote, attention to this ongoing production heightens therapists' responsive involvement or discursive reflexivity—the discursive cousin to Tomm's notion of reflexivity suggested in our first initial quote (i.e., activating the reflexivity among meanings within preexisting belief systems).

Tomm (1987b) portrayed reflexive questioning as an aspect of interventive interviewing, an empowering conceptual "posture" oriented toward fostering clients as autonomous agents of change—toward "enabling clients to generate new patterns of cognition and behavior on their own" (p. 4). Arguably, fostering clients' autonomy and self-determination is not just more effective but also more ethical, as compared to therapists persistently advancing *their* meanings and proposals when clients consistently display or convey reluctance to take them up (see, e.g., CPA, 2000, Principle I). It is our hope that our brief discursive analysis helps make this reflexive conversational process more visible—it is an observable, researchable, teachable, and learnable activity. We offered an alternative, discursive conception of client agency, presently marginalized in the field, which can complement a more conventional understanding of agency as a key variable accounting for positive therapy outcomes (e.g., Asay & Lambert, 1999; Bohart & Wade, 2013; Gonzalez, 2016). A conception of client agency and other preferred client accounts as discursively or interactionally constituted may be useful to practitioners, particularly discursive, social constructionist practitioners who see social interaction and language use in therapy as constitutive (rather than reflective) of clients' subjectivities and relationships. Rather than seeing clients' agency (or other preferred client self-understandings) as internal and stable, we offered a perspective on agency as a practical, situated accomplishment.

Our hope in writing this chapter was to highlight the discursive basis of reflexive questions: how lines of talk (attributional work) are invited through reflexive questions that subsequently involve responsive attributional work to arrive at mutually preferred answers to those invitations. We encourage therapists to adopt a discursive orientation in their work with clients that envisions therapy as discourse. Through discursive psychological inquiry, the sequentiality and nuance of therapeutic actions can become more available to awareness to be employed in the service of therapeutic goals.

Acknowledgment Work on this chapter was supported by funding received from CONICYT, Fondecyt Program No. 11150198.

References

Anderson, H. (1997). *Conversation, language, and possibilities: A postmodern approach to therapy*. New York, NY: Basic Books.

Andersen, T. (1987). The reflecting team: Dialogue and meta-dialogue in clinical work. *Family Process, 26*, 415–428.

Asay, T. P., & Lambert, M. J. (1999). The empirical case for the common factors in therapy: Quantitative findings. In A. Hubble, B. Duncan, & S. Miller (Eds.), *The heart and soul of change: What works in therapy* (pp. 23–55). Washington, DC: American Psychological Association.

Avdi, E. (2005). Negotiating a pathological identity in the clinical dialogue: Discourse analysis of a family therapy. *Psychology and Psychotherapy: Theory, Research and Practice, 78*(4), 493–511.

Berger, P. L., & Luckmann, T. (1991). *The social construction of reality: A treatise in the sociology of knowledge*. London: Penguin.

Bohart, A. C., & Tallman, K. (2010). Clients: The neglected common factor in psychotherapy. In B. L. Duncan, S. D. Miller, B. E. Wampold, & M. A.

Hubble (Eds.), *The heart and soul of change: Delivering what works in therapy* (pp. 83–111). Washington, DC: American Psychological Association.
Bohart, A. C., & Wade, A. G. (2013). The client in psychotherapy. In M. Lambert (Ed.), *Bergin and Garfield's handbook of psychotherapy and behavior change* (6th ed., pp. 219–257). Hoboken, NJ: Wiley.
Buber, M. (1970). *I and Thou*. New York, NY: Charles Scribner's Sons.
Buttny, R. (1990). Blame–account sequences in therapy: The negotiation of relational meanings. *Semiotica, 78*(3–4), 219–248.
Canadian Psychological Association. (2000). *Canadian code of ethics for psychologists* (3rd. ed.). Ottawa, ON: Author Retrieved from http://www.cpa.ca/docs/File/Ethics/cpa_code_2000_eng_jp_jan2014.pdf
Combs, G., & Freedman, J. (2012). Narrative, poststructuralism, and social justice: Current practices in narrative therapy. *The Counseling Psychologist, 40*(7), 1033–1060.
De Jong, P., & Berg, I. K. (2002). *Interviewing for solutions* (2nd ed.). Pacific Grove, CA: Brooks/Cole.
De Shazer, S. (1984). The death of resistance. *Family Process, 23*(1), 11–17.
Dreier, O. (2015). Interventions in everyday lives: How clients use psychotherapy outside their sessions. *European Journal of Psychotherapy & Counselling, 17*(2), 114–128.
Edwards, D. (1997). *Discourse and cognition*. London, UK: Sage.
Edwards, D. (1999). Emotion discourse. *Culture & Psychology, 5*(3), 271–291.
Edwards, D. (2005). Discursive psychology. In K. L. Fitch & R. E. Sanders (Eds.), *Handbook of language and social interaction* (pp. 257–273). Hillsdale, NJ: Erlbaum.
Edwards, D., & Potter, J. (1992). *Discursive psychology*. London: Sage.
Freedman, J., & Combs, G. (1996). *Narrative therapy: The social construction of preferred realities*. New York: Norton.
Gadamer, H. G. (2004). *Truth and method* (J. Weinsheimer & D. G. Marshall, Trans., 2nd Rev. ed.). New York, NY: Continuum.
Gendlin, E. T. (1996). *Focusing-oriented psychotherapy: A manual of the experiential method*. New York, NY: Guilford Press.
Gonzalez, D. M. (2016). Client variables and psychotherapy outcomes. In D. J. Cain, K. Keenan, & S. Rubin (Eds.), *Humanistic psychotherapies: Handbook of research and practice* (2nd ed.). Washington, DC: American Psychological Association.
Greenberg, L. S., & Pinsoff, W. (1986). *The psychotherapeutic process: A research handbook*. New York, NY: Guilford Press.

Hayano, K. (2013). Question design in conversation. In J. Sidnell & T. Stivers (Eds.), *The handbook of conversation analysis* (pp. 395–414). Malden, MA: Wiley-Blackwell.

Hepburn, A., & Potter, J. (2012). Crying and crying responses. In A. Peräkylä & M.-L. Sorjonen (Eds.), *Emotions in interaction* (pp. 195–211). New York, NY: Oxford University Press.

Hepburn, A., & Wiggins, S. (Eds.). (2005). Developments in discursive psychology. *Discourse & Society, 16*(5), 595–601.

Heritage, J. (2013). Epistemics in conversation. In J. Sidnell & T. Stivers (Eds.), *The handbook of conversation analysis* (pp. 370–394). Malden, MA: Wiley-Blackwell.

Jefferson, G. (1984). Notes on a systematic deployment of the acknowledgement tokens 'yah' and 'mm hm'. *Papers in Linguistics, 17*, 197–216.

Jefferson, G. (1991). List-construction as a task and resource. In G. Psathas (Ed.), *Interactional competence* (pp. 63–92). New York: Irvington Publishers.

Lindstrom, A., & Sorjonen, M.-L. (2013). Affiliation in conversation. In J. Sidnell & T. Stivers (Eds.), *The handbook of conversation analysis* (pp. 350–369). Malden, MA: Wiley-Blackwell.

Lock, A., & Strong, T. (Eds.). (2012). *Discursive perspectives in therapeutic practice*. Oxford, UK: Oxford University Press.

MacMartin, C. (2008). Resisting optimistic questions in narrative and solution-focused therapies. In A. Peräkylä, C. Antaki, S. Vehviläinen, & I. Leudar (Eds.), *Conversation analysis and psychotherapy* (pp. 80–99). New York, NY: CUP.

O'Reilly, M. (2014). Blame and accountability in family therapy: Making sense of therapeutic spaces discursively. [Special issue]. *Qualitative Psychology, 1*(2), 163–177.

Orlinsky, D. E., Ronnestad, M. H., & Willutzki, U. (2004). Fifty years of psychotherapy process-outcome research: Continuity and change. In J. Clarkin, K. Levi, A. Bergin, & S. Garfield (Eds.), *Handbook of psychotherapy and behavior change* (5th ed., pp. 307–390). Hoboken, NJ: Wiley.

Paré, D. (2012). *The practice of collaborative counseling and psychotherapy: Developing skills in culturally mindful helping*. Los Angeles, CA: Sage.

Patrika, P., & Tseliou, E. (2016). Blame, responsibility and systemic neutrality: A discourse analysis methodology to the study of family therapy problem talk. *Journal of Family Therapy, 38*(4), 467–490.

Peräkylä, A. (1995). *AIDS counselling: Institutional interaction and clinical practice*. Cambridge: Cambridge University Press.

Pomerantz, A. (1986). Extreme case formulations: A way of legitimizing claims. *Human Studies, 9*(2–3), 219–229. https://doi.org/10.1007/BF00148128
Pomerantz, A., & Heritage, J. (2013). Preference. In J. Sidnell & T. Stivers (Eds.), *Handbook of conversation analysis* (pp. 210–228). Hoboken, NJ: Wiley-Blackwell Press.
Potter, J. (1996). *Representing reality*. London: Sage.
Potter, J. (2010). Contemporary discursive psychology: Issues, prospects and Corcoran's awkward ontology. *British Journal of Social Psychology, 49*, 691–701.
Potter, J., & Hepburn, A. (2007). Discursive psychology: Mind and reality in practice. In *Language, discourse and social psychology* (pp. 160–180). London: Palgrave Macmillan.
Prochaska, J. O., DiClemente, C. C., & Norcross, J. C. (1992). In search of how people change: Applications to addictive behaviors. *American Psychologist, 47*(9), 1102–1114.
Raymond, G. (2003). Grammar and social organization: Yes/no interrogatives and the structure of responding. *American Sociological Review, 68*(6), 939–967. https://doi.org/10.2307/1519752
Shotter, J. (2008). *Conversational realities revisited: Life, language, body and world*. Chagrin Falls, OH: Taos Institute Publications.
Speer, S. A. (2012). Hypothetical questions: A comparative analysis and implications for 'applied' versus 'basic' conversation analysis. *Research on Language and Social Interaction, 45*(4), 352–374.
Stancombe, J., & White, S. (2005). Cause and responsibility: Towards an interactional understanding of blaming and 'neutrality'in family therapy. *Journal of Family Therapy, 27*(4), 330–351.
Strong, T. (2007). Accomplishments in social constructionist counseling: Micro-analytic and retrospective analyses. *Qualitative Research in Psychology, 4*(1–2), 85–105.
Sutherland, O. A., Sametband, I., Gaete, J., Couture, S. J., & Strong, T. (2013). Conversational perspective of therapeutic outcomes: The importance of preference in the development of discourse. *Counselling and Psychotherapy Research, 13*(3), 220–226.
Te Molder, H. (2015). Discursive psychology. In K. Tracy, C. Ilie, & T. Sandel (Eds.), *The international encyclopedia of language and social interaction* (pp. 1–11). Boston, MA: Wiley.
Tileagă, C., & Stokoe, E. (Eds.). (2016). *Discursive psychology: Classic and contemporary issues*. New York: Routledge.

Tomm, K. (1987a). Interventive interviewing: Part I. Strategizing as a fourth guideline for the therapist. *Family Process, 26*, 2–13. https://doi.org/10.1111/j.1545-5300.1987.00003.x
Tomm, K. (1987b). Interventive interviewing: Part II. Reflexive questioning as a means to enable self-healing. *Family Process, 26*, 153–183. https://doi.org/10.1111/j.1545-5300.1987.00167.x
Tomm, K. (1988). Interventive interviewing: Part III. Intending to ask lineal, circular, reflexive and strategic questions? *Family Process, 27*, 1–15. https://doi.org/10.1111/j.1545-5300.1988.00001.x
Vehviläinen, S. (2008). Identifying and managing resistance in psychoanalytic interaction. In A. Peräkylä, C. Antaki, S. Vehviläinen, & I. Leudar (Eds.), *Conversation analysis and psychotherapy* (pp. 120–138). Cambridge: Cambridge University Press.
Watzlawick, P., Beavin, J., & Jackson, D. (1967). *Pragmatics of human communication*. New York, NY: W. W. Norton.
Weingarten, K. (1992). A consideration of intimate and non-intimate interactions in therapy. *Family Process, 31*(1), 45–59. https://doi.org/10.1111/j.1545-5300.1992.00045.x
White, M. (2003). Narrative practice and community assignments. *International Journal of Narrative Therapy and Community Work, 2*(1), 17–56.
White, M. (2007). *Maps of narrative practice*. New York, NY: WW Norton & Company.
White, M., & Epston, D. (1990). *Narrative means to therapeutic ends*. New York, NY: WW Norton & Company.
Wiggins, S. (2017). *Discursive psychology: Theory, method and application*. London: Sage.
Wittgenstein, L. (1953). *Philosophical investigations*. Oxford: Blackwell.

7

Transforming Gender Discourse in Couple Therapy: Researching Intersections of Societal Discourse, Emotion, and Interaction

Carmen Knudson-Martin, Jessica ChenFeng, Aimee Galick, Elsie Lobo, Sarah K. Samman, and Kirstee Williams

C. Knudson-Martin (✉)
Graduate School of Education and Counseling, Lewis and Clark College, Portland, OR, USA
e-mail: carmen@lclark.edu

J. ChenFeng
California State University, Northridge, CA, USA
e-mail: Jessica.chen@csun.edu

A. Galick
Government of Alberta, Edmonton, AB, Canada
e-mail: agalick@llu.edu

E. Lobo
Loma Linda University, Loma Linda, CA, USA
e-mail: elobo@llu.edu

S. K. Samman
Alliant International University, San Diego, CA, USA
e-mail: sarah.samman@alliant.edu

O. Smoliak, T. Strong (eds.), *Therapy as Discourse*, The Language of Mental Health,
https://doi.org/10.1007/978-3-319-93067-1_7

Socio-Emotional Relationship Therapy (SERT) is a critical social constructionist approach that seeks to transform power inequities and promote relational possibilities based on mutual support and justice (Knudson-Martin, 2016). As a form of critical praxis (Collins & Bilge, 2016), SERT practitioners believe that therapy is a sociopolitical activity in which therapists conceptualize symptoms within systems of power and privilege and position their work to challenge and undo limiting or oppressive dominant standards (Baber, 2009; Kahn & Monk, 2017; Lorber, 2005). The approach, which involves three concurrent aspects of discursive process: societal discourse (Foucault, 1973), emotion (Wetherell, 2012), and patterned interaction (Bourdieu, 1986; McDowell, 2015), evolved out of action research that began at Loma Linda University in Southern California in 2008 (see Knudson-Martin et al., 2015).

A team of doctoral students and faculty met weekly to observe live couple and family therapy sessions and systematically study our work. This participatory action approach enabled synergy between critical inquiry and clinical practice, with analysis of power at the center of each (Collins & Bilge, 2016; Wodak & Meyer, 2016). We began with a definition of discourse as sets of shared social meanings that operate at multiple levels of abstraction from individual to institutional (Fairclough, 2016; Krolekke & Sorensen, 2006). In this view, discourses both construct social action and are constructed by it. As practicing relationship therapists, we are interested in the dialectic between social discourses at the societal and interpersonal levels; how do societal discourses at the institutional level position therapy and how may therapy contribute to transforming them? As clinicians, we find it helpful to emphasize discourses as having constitutive action outside the individual (Wodak & Meyer, 2016). As critical theorists, we are constantly balancing between very real societal inequities that social practices maintain, and developing strategies that begin to undo them.

In order to identify themes and determine how categories of discursive practices theoretically connect with each other in embodied use, we

K. Williams
Lee University, Cleveland, TN, USA
e-mail: kirsteewilliams@leeuniversity.edu

applied qualitative methods outside the usual discursive approaches. The first phases involved developing a set of SERT competencies through a process similar to the consensual qualitative approach (Hill, Thompson, & Williams, 1997). This was an iterative activity in which team members responded to evolving themes until everyone's experience was incorporated and we reached a shared understanding. Then we studied specific aspects of these competencies and refined them. As the model solidified, we drew on grounded theory analyses of videotaped sessions to understand pieces that appeared particularly challenging or important.

In this chapter, we describe the discursive framework that guides SERT and show how we used a variety of qualitative methods to understand and explain the clinical work. Though the SERT approach addresses intersections of all social locations, here we emphasize clinical processes around gendered power.

The SERT Framework

As a critical social constructionist approach, SERT attends to the intersections between patterned social structures, societal discourse, emotion, and power (Baber, 2009; Wetherell, 2012). Personal experience, including the physiological, cannot be separated from societal context and yet people also have agency in what they do; that is, societal discourses do not fully determine individual action (Gergen, 2006; Lorber, 2005). Though there are always multiple potential discourses within any context (Winslade, 2009), discursive practices position everyone in relation to dominant sociocultural discourses in some way (Davies & Harré, 1990; Harré, Moghaddam, Cairnie, Rothbart, & Sabat, 2009). These dominant discourses maintain and reflect interests of the powerful (Foucault, 1973). SERT therapists intentionally position their work to interrupt and transform inequitable societal discourses as they play out in the clinical encounter; that is, they are purposeful about which societal discourses their reflections, queries, and interventions support or invite. Positioning may include resistance to dominant discourses and/or draw on marginalized discourses (Garcia, Košutic, & McDowell, 2015).

Emotion is how we register societal relationship in our bodies (Knudson-Martin & Huenergardt, 2010; Wetherell, 2012). According to Burkitt (2014), "feelings and emotions form our embodied, mindful sense" of on-going patterned relationships (p. 15). They are part of the discursive process by which people orient to each other, create, reproduce, and—potentially—transform themselves and each other. Social meaning, relationship patterns, and visceral experience are "intra-twined" (Shotter, 2014, p. 111). SERT attends to in-the-moment affective experiential process as a way to engage and transform discursive process.

Our bodies read the power context of every social relationship, which becomes part of perception and affects communication (Wetherell, 2012). Inequitable societal power processes create inequities in how people notice, respond, attend, and accommodate each other (Knudson-Martin, 2013). Stereotypic gender discourses invite men to take a dominant discursive position in which they expect to be attended to, but are less likely to notice and attend to their partners. They place responsibility for maintaining relationship on women and discourage men from vulnerability or opening themselves to influence. If heterosexual partners do not resist these gender discourses, power differences are embodied in their relationships.

SERT therapists counter power differences by working from a relationship model that emphasizes mutual vulnerability, mutual attunement, mutual influence, and shared relational responsibility (Knudson-Martin & Huenergardt, 2010). In other words, we bring a counter discourse to the clinical dialogue. Therapists do not impose this discourse in a didactic way; they use the framework to guide questions and in-the-moment clinical process. The emphasis on mutuality makes SERT applicable to all relationships; however, the research included in this chapter focuses on heterosexual couples.

To advance the SERT approach and inform clinical decisions, we draw on practice-based evidence (St. George, Wulff, & Strong, 2014), using a variety of process-oriented methods. In the sections that follow we describe methods and key findings from four studies in our on-going action research. The first is a grounded theory analysis of how dominant gender discourses influence therapeutic process. The second also used grounded theory to explain how to relationally engage men in session. The third is a task analysis of how therapists facilitate mutuality in cases of infidelity. We conclude with a narrative case analysis that details the interplay between discursive positioning and neurobiological discourse. All help delineate the socio-emotional processes involved as couples reposition and transform how they perform societal discourses regarding gender. We view all categories of people referenced in these studies (e.g., wife, male, heterosexual, etc.) as socially constructed.

How Gender Discourse Practices Position Couple Therapy

Our first project was to identify how gender discourses are present and influence in-session couple therapy processes. We used a grounded theory analysis (ChenFeng & Galick, 2015) based on 23 transcripts of couple therapy sessions conducted *prior* to the development of SERT. The sample included 19 heterosexual client couples and 17 therapists, with diversity across age, race, and ethnicity. Therapists were advanced doctoral students and two licensed Marriage and Family Therapy (MFT) professors. They described a variety of theoretical modalities, for example, narrative, solution-focused, Bowen family systems, structural therapy, and feminist. Six sessions were with co-therapists with one female, one male; 11 sessions were with solo female therapists; two were with a male therapist. The gender of the therapists in four sessions was not identified.

Authors Jessica ChenFeng and Aimee Galick began their analysis at the start of their doctoral programs when they had little awareness of how gender and other societal context affected clinical issues (ChenFeng & Galick, 2015). They started with a broad question about how gender, culture, and societal power were present in therapy sessions and little presumed knowledge about the subject. Grounded theory methodology provided a systematic process to engage with transcript data on a line-by-line basis, naming what they saw with no pre-determined categories (Charmaz, 2014). They then looked for similarities and differences in the identified codes and considered how these categories were connected. This enabled them to understand what might account for variations in the observed processes; that is, develop grounded theory about the discursive practices involved.

At the beginning Jessica and Aimee tried to code examples of all kinds of sociocultural discourses. They found that gender discourses seemed especially salient, and decided to focus specifically on how gender discourses influenced what was happening. Three gender discourses appeared primary to practice in almost all transcripts, so they focused their coding more explicitly on the discursive processes associated with them:

- Men should be the authority
- Women should be responsible for relationships
- Women should protect men from shame

Most of the time the dialogue among all participants—male and female, therapists and clients—reinforced and maintained the discourses, but sometimes therapists engaged in ways that countered them.

Actions that Reinforce Gender Discourse

Spotting discursive actions that reinforced gender discourse was difficult at first. Jessica and Aimee had been socialized not to see them. "We had to listen very, very carefully and pay deliberate attention so we could hear what we typically did not notice" (ChenFeng & Galick, 2015, p. 46). Actions that reinforced gender discourses were subtle; for example, who questions were directed to, who answered which kinds of questions, whose construction of the story was followed, which experiences and perspectives were validated, who was asked to change, what partners were asked to change, and what the presenting problem became.

Privileging Men's Experiences

Again and again, men's experiences and views became privileged and women's experiences minimized by her partner and the therapist. When the male client answered a question, therapists often automatically took up his view as *the* concern without tending to the female client's experience. This reinforced the discourse that men should be the authority and women should defer to them. Sounds outdated, doesn't it? Yet it happened regularly.

In one session a wife tried to talk about her experience of losing their baby before term. Her husband went back and forth between medical causes for the loss and blaming his wife for their marital problems. He often spoke over her and cut her off. By not interrupting this dynamic, the therapist reinforced the gender discourse that men are the authority. When the therapist eventually redirected the conversation by asking, "How is your relationship now?" the wife answered, "It's still rocky." The therapist immediately sought the husband's view. The husband took up the discourse that women are responsible for the relationship, placing blame for their problems on her "cycle." The therapist again reinforced these discourses by following the husband's version of the story.

Expecting Women to Accommodate

Therapists regularly asked women to change. In the session described above, the therapist first asked the husband "what he needed from his wife during this difficult time." He responded, "If her perceptions change, I think that alone will pretty much take care of everything," again placing responsibility on his wife. The therapist again aligned with dominant gender discourse, asking the husband to expand upon his needs and helping the wife reflect upon how she could change. "The therapist never asked the wife what she needed from her husband or validated her experience around the loss" (ChenFeng & Galick, 2015, p. 47).

Protecting Men from Shame

The expectation that "women should protect men from shame," repeated across sessions, enacted the idea that women are responsible for relationships. We saw therapists reinforcing this discourse when they did not address or follow up on female concerns and instead focused on what she was doing to improve the relationship. When one woman said, "everything is good [in the relationship] as long as I don't have any complaints," the therapist changed the subject rather than counteracting the discourse by encouraging her to explore the issues she might wish to address (ChenFeng & Galick, 2015, p. 47). Therapist actions like this reinforced societal expectations that women should protect men from shame and blame, even at their own expense.

Countering Dominant Gender Discourse

Once Jessica and Aimee saw how systematically therapeutic dialogue reinforced dominant gender discourse across sessions, they brought this finding back to the larger research group. We became very interested in learning how therapists could counter gender discourse. Jessica and Aimee went back to transcripts to look for exceptions. In grounded theory explaining exceptions can help to identify paths for transformation. This happened when therapists voiced or acknowledged alternative discourses. For example, they validated men for relational actions and women for expressing their needs or framed relationship patterns as part of societal discourse:

> (to husband) You were present, you were listening, you were attending, you were there, and as you processed your thoughts, you also gave [her] the space to process hers … you could have just given up … and checked out. (ChenFeng & Galick, 2015, p. 48)

This study clarified for us that in order to promote relationships that equitably support each partner, we have to engage male partners in ways that counter the dominating gender discourses. We set out to learn how best to facilitate men's engagement.

How Therapists Influence Male Relational Engagement

Our group observed that when men engaged in therapy they tended to focus on their own experiences and perceptions and did not demonstrate what we termed "relational engagement." Helping men develop and operate from a more relational discourse was key to success. In order to develop a clearer picture of how to do this work, Sarah Samman took the lead in a grounded theory study.

Method

As is usual in grounded theory research, the sample was selected to best answer our theoretical questions (Charmaz, 2014). We identified and transcribed video segments of therapy with highly distressed heterosexual couples in which male partners appeared caught in an individualistic approach to relationship. They exemplified Loscocco and Walzer's (2013) analysis that marriage culture in the US is organized around male independence and individuality, while women carry responsibility for the relationship. We studied 28 couple therapy sessions with 11 couples comprising a variety of ages, ethnicities, and educational levels. Therapists were from diverse backgrounds and included nine Marriage and Family Therapy doctoral students and two faculty supervisors. All used SERT to guide the sessions.

Sarah began with line-by-line coding. She used no pre-determined categories and instead labeled what she saw happening based on our interest in how to relationally engage men in therapy: For example, when a man said, "I get nervous … but in the end, I feel better … because I know she feels better," this was coded as "positive experience of attending to wife's comfort" (Samman & Knudson-Martin, 2015, p. 83). Initial codes were grouped together and brought to a larger group to consider how these categories explained whether men took a more relationally engaged position. The final analysis identified a set of five therapist actions that helped transform male engagement from individualism discourse to a relational stance.

Findings

The following worked together to facilitate and sustain each successful transformation: (1) attend to male's sociocultural context, (2) validate male's relational intent, followed immediately with, (3) highlight the impact of male's behavior on the female partner, (4) punctuate alternative relational interactions, and (5) demonstrate persistent therapist leadership (Samman & Knudson-Martin, 2015).

Attend to Sociocultural Context

Attending to sociocultural context appeared preliminary to the rest of the transformation process and occurred regularly over time. A male client explained the value of this:

> Well, whoever I become, including this person who detaches, is in response to this world in which I live. Being aware of it is helpful and recognizing sometimes the fact that I'm doing it ... see how it might have [harmed as well as] benefited me [as a Black male] at times. (Samman & Knudson-Martin, 2015, p. 84)

Validate Male's Relational Intent and Highlight Impact on Female

It was important to validate men's relational intent. However, this needed to be followed *immediately* with highlighting the impact of their behavior on their partners (Samman & Knudson-Martin, 2015, p. 85–86):

> Therapist: I really get that she's important to you and that you feel compelled to stay in charge because you love her and want her to get the best treatment and be healthy.
>
> Howard: Yeah, I do want her to be around longer. Much longer.

The therapist followed validation with questions about the impact of Howard's behavior on his partner:

> Therapist: I can also understand that you're used to being in charge and I'm wondering how you think being in charge of her treatment impacts her?
>
> Howard [to partner]: When you get scared, I get scared and I think you struggle with my way of doing things.
>
> Therapist: What do you think she needs from you right now?
>
> Howard [to partner]: I think you need to have a voice in your treatment.

Punctuate Alternative Relational Interactions

When men engaged relationally, therapists punctuated this new discursive position and connected it to positive relational effects.

Therapist: Mathew, you responded to her honesty with active listening … [Looking at Mary] Would it be right to assume you felt heard?
Mary: Absolutely. I did actually. It felt really good. I felt valued.

This kind of systemic/circular questioning about one's effect on others helps develop relational, "we-oriented" discourse.

Demonstrate Persistent Therapist Leadership

Enacting new relational discourse required persistent therapist leadership over time, meaning that therapists took active steps to bring the less aware relational discourse into the clinical conversation.

Therapist: … I'm curious though, I haven't heard about relating to Lena at an emotional level.
Miguel: I'm not relating on an emotional level right now. But I would like to act differently. I want to.
Therapist: What would that look like?
Miguel: Not talking from my head all the time.
Therapist: What would that feel like?
Miguel: It would feel real, more connected. I want to connect with her more. (Samman & Knudson-Martin, 2015, p. 87)

This grounded theory analysis was invaluable in clarifying specific steps that therapists could take to help male partners move from an "I" oriented discourse to enacting a more "we" focused relational discourse. In a related study, our group also wanted to consider how to frame symptoms and outcomes within clinical discourses that value equity and mutuality. We decided to focus on infidelity.

From Inequality to Mutuality Following Infidelity

Kirstee Williams and Carmen Knudson-Martin (2013) used grounded theory methods to analyze how the literature on treatment for infidelity addressed gender and power. They found that authors spoke *as though* partners were equal, and in so doing, overlooked power processes. They did not consider how the relational meaning of an affair may differ depending on whether the affair was an attempt to equalize an imbalance of power or was based on entitlement associated with a dominant power position. In response to this finding, Kirstee developed a model for treating infidelity based on SERT (Williams, 2011) and used task analysis to refine the model (Williams, Galick, Knudson-Martin, & Huenergardt, 2013).

Method

A task analysis identifies clinically meaningful "change events," that is, client-therapist sequences, and builds mini-theory around how this change occurs (Greenberg, 2007). It requires that researchers already be knowledgeable about the conceptual framework and able to interpret clinical actions through that lens. Kirstee and her research team set about detailing the processes through which societal discourses supporting power imbalances were transformed. They targeted mutual support as the end goal and began by identifying a sample of change events in which couples successfully demonstrated it, that is, moments when mutual attunement, mutual influence, shared vulnerability, and shared relational responsibility occurred. In this way, we could identify in-the-moment outcomes along the way to larger discursive change.

Thirteen examples of successful change events and seven unsuccessful ones were drawn from 15 videotaped couple therapy sessions representing five client couples and six therapists. Couples were heterosexual, with four men and one woman committing the infidelity. MFT doctoral students who had received training in SERT conducted the therapy. Couples and therapists were ethnically diverse. Five of the therapists were female and one was male. All therapists in successful change events were women.

Our analysis resulted in a model with five core components. Two of the components—(1) attention to power dynamics and (2) attunement to gender context—provided the foundation for the three remaining components: (3) creating space for alternate gender discourses, (4) pursuing relational responsibility of the more powerful partner, and (5) deepening experience of mutual support (Williams et al., 2013, p. 289).

Attention to Power Dynamics

Two strategies facilitated therapists' ability to attend to power dynamics: (1) strong leadership and (2) not relating to the couple as though they are equal (Williams et al., 2013). Therapists who attended to power dynamics avoided language that suggested partners were equal, such as "both of you." They attended to how gender discourses organized each person's contribution to relationship maintenance, for example, by giving voice to unspoken gender discourse: "Is it hard for you to hear that you made her scared?" (Williams et al., 2013, p. 290).

Attunement to Gender Context

Therapists in successful change events also connected gender discourses with power processes. In this example, the therapist identified the male partner's gender discourse around competence, then connected it to his ability to hear his wife: "...so as she shares her needs ... just try and really hear what they are and not get caught up in I messed up again" (Williams et al., 2013, p. 291). In unsuccessful change events, the affair was discussed only as a relationship problem and not connected to contextual issues of gender and power. When therapists voiced clients' unspoken gendered experiences, the couples appeared receptive to alternate gender discourses that would foster mutuality.

Creating Space for Alternate Gender Discourses

It was not enough to simply identify stereotypic gender patterns. Therapists in successful change events actively created space for alternate gender discourses by highlighting and privileging new ways of being in a relationship beyond scripted gender training (Williams et al., 2013). Because gender discourses keep peace by encouraging female accommodation, a primary task in facilitating alternate ways of relating (i.e., mutuality) was to create space for the woman's voice and support male partners in taking in her reality. Therapists do this by attuning to the female partner's sense of reality and facilitating the male partner's attunement toward her. Helping the powerful partner express vulnerability is also a necessary part of this process.

Pursue Relational Responsibility of Powerful Partner

A critical choice point in transforming how gender relationships are enacted is putting relational responsibility on the powerful partner. In the example below (Williams et al., 2013, p. 293), in which the husband had the affair, the therapist actively facilitated his attunement to her by asking him to inquire about his wife's experience. Notice his difficulty focusing on her and how the therapist persisted in engaging him with her:

> Therapist: Do you think that surprise would make her teary? So, ask her what the feeling was?
> Husband: Well, I know my tears were of joy.
> Therapist: What about hers?
> Husband: Well, she pretty much answered that.
> Therapist: Just ask her.
> Husband: [To wife] were your tears of joy?
> Wife: Well, yea, because like you said, you missed me.

Expanding Experience of Mutual Support

In successful change events, therapists helped partners counteract sociocultural gender discourses by returning to and expanding upon new, more mutual experiences—again and again. They provided a form of leadership similar to Sutherland, Turner, and Dienhart's (2013) notion of responsive persistence; while staying close to client experience and preferences, therapists held responsibility for bringing discourses of mutuality from the margins to the center. At the same time, we were aware that clinical discourses around neurobiology are also often used to promote shared relational engagement (Fishbane, 2013; Strong, 2017). We wondered what we might see when we observed SERT re-positioning practices through a neurobiological lens.

The Neurobiology of Re-positioning

Neurobiological discourse suggests that when people relate to each other based on social discourses, brain development is implicated; that is, synaptic connections are triggered and retriggered (Cozolinio, 2016; Siegel, 2012). From a discursive point of view, emotions, power, and social discourse are all temporally and situationally intertwined as "body and body sensations are fused with social meanings in the patterned relational weavings of social encounters" (Burkitt, 2014, p. 169). In these intersubjective socio-emotional moments, societal discourse and power relations are embodied (Wetherell, 2012). This is a relational process in which the impetus for change resides in social interaction (Strong, 2017). Elsie Lobo took the lead in studying how neurobiological discourses may inform our understanding of what happens when therapists position their work to counter constraining discursive practices (Lobo & Knudson-Martin, 2015).

Method

We decided that in-depth narrative analysis (Riessman, 2008) of one case over time would allow us to explore new territory in integrating the discursive processes of positioning theory with experiential attention to the in-the-moment processes between the couple and with the therapist. Elsie selected four sessions of a case in which Carmen Knudson-Martin (female) and Douglas Huenergardt (male), founders of SERT, worked with a Euro-American heterosexual couple married for 26 years. The couple entered therapy locked into stereotypic gender patterns. Earlier in their marriage the wife had liked the security of a strong male provider. Now she had begun to resist the discourse. The husband responded to her anger with escalating anger until she accommodated or withdrew into depression.

Elsie began by viewing the video and transcripts in detail, noting what happened from three perspectives: positioning theory, gender and power processes, and observations based on the interpersonal neurobiology literature. Then she conferred with Carmen and other members of the research team to consider how the identified processes worked together in therapy. They adapted three previously identified stages of SERT (Knudson-Martin & Huenergardt, 2015) to fit with the understandings.

Findings

The narrative analysis identified clinical processes similar to previous studies and added an experiential, neurobiological lens from which to view the SERT clinical sequence.

Dimension I—Awareness of Gender Inequity and Clinical Positioning

Awareness of societal discourse enabled clients to see choice about how they positioned themselves in relationship to social discourse. Neurobiological discourse posits that when information is conscious, it is more stable and more available for the neural reorganization implicated as discursive practices change (Siegel, 2012). This helps people respond beyond automatic reflex (Cozolinio, 2016). In the sessions, the male client came to an awareness of the impact of gender discourse on his response to his wife, "It is my arrogance, I guess … it's not even that I'm trying to be the knight in shining armor, I'm trying to tell her."

Recognition that clients are being constrained to perform gendered roles enabled the therapist to empathize with their experience while remaining positioned against the inequities. *Empathy* reduced clients' fear, which is said to also stimulate neuroplastic processes involved in change (Cozolinio, 2016). When the male client said, "I never planned for those [aggressive] feelings to come back, they just do," the therapist was able to empathically respond, "I know. You hate those feelings … this has to the potential to sabotage [your relationship] and we don't want that to happen."

Dimension II—Experiential Processes That Renegotiate Power Positions

Countering socially prescribed interactions was facilitated when each partner *felt safe* to risk performing behaviors outside of their usual discursive position. According to neurobiological discourse, creating a safe environment stimulates social engagement at the neurochemical level and helps partners be receptive to each other (Porges, 2009). The therapist worked to *be with* the dominant male partner as he learned to create safety for his wife, "What would be comforting for her … [to be] able to talk about it with you and feel as if you're safe?" The husband seemed to feel supported and able to engage, responding, "yeah, that was the word I was just going to use, that she's safe."

Interrupting power provided the opportunity to experientially practice new, preferred discourses. From a neurological perspective, these practices promoted development of new neuronal networks to overtake the old ones (Fishbane, 2013). For example, when the husband raised an issue regarding his wife and her father, the wife quietly said she did not want to talk about it. The husband persisted. The therapist interrupted this power dynamic, "Wait a minute … [to wife] is this something you want to talk about?" The therapists then helped the male client challenge dominant male discourse by *attuning* to both his own process and to hers. Therapist to husband, "How do you know what [wife] needs? How do you figure that out?" Husband, "Well, because I can see her pain …" Therapist: "So you imagine that would be painful?" Husband (softly), "Yeah, it would." Focusing on the mental state of each other helped neurologically embody mutual attunement.

Dimension III—Practice of New Positioning in Relationship

Though clients were not yet free of all discursive constraints, they began to interact more consistently with their preferred, more just, and mutually supportive position. These new interactions reinforced the connections between the implicated neural pathways. In neurobiological discourse, those that do not get actuated "can die away" (Siegel, 2012, p. 253). In this example, when the therapist helped the wife reinforce challenges to the dominant gender discourse, new neural pathways were invited. Therapist: "So what did it take on your part to do what you felt was right?" Wife: "I just had to deal with it … and come to my own conclusions." Therapist: "[In the past] you were saying 'if I don't do it his way, I wonder if I'll get flack.' Did those worries come up for you or did those worries somehow not have much power?" Wife: "They were there … I didn't give him the power to influence my decision." Therapist: "So worry was there, but you…" Wife: "I just had to do what I felt was right."

This study helped us conceptualize how new discourses become physiologically embodied and how the transformative process engages neurobiological systems. In particular, the neurobiological discourse highlighted three important relational components: awareness, safety (through empathy and attending to power), and practice.

Conclusion

The studies reported in this chapter were based on the idea that discursive processes include acting and feeling, as well as thinking and speaking (Shotter, 2014; Wetherell, 2012). While not usually considered discourse analyses, we have shown how grounded theory and task analysis enabled us to detail clinical strategies that effectively help clients re-position themselves in relation to dominant gender discourses. We were able to fine-tune a practice-based clinical sequence for Socio-Emotional Relationship Therapy that can be taught and evaluated. Three interconnected phases are involved: (1) positioning—attuning to sociocultural emotion and discourse and exposing relational consequences of power inequities; (2) interrupting—shifting sociocultural discourses in in-the-moment relational power processes; and (3) practicing—envisioning new mutuality, enacting increased options for shared responsibility, and reinforcing these new practices.

This approach can help clients recognize alternatives within systems of systems so as to intentionally position themselves to create more just relationships and navigate the influences of societal inequities in their lives

(McDowell, Knudson-Martin, & Bermudez, 2018). These kinds of micro-level interventions within couple and family relationships are also a political intervention at the societal level, making small, but not inconsequential, advances across all levels of social action.

These findings open new areas for research in the *how* of practice aimed at transforming inequitable gender/societal discourses. We need to discover what enables clinicians to recognize societal discourses in client stories and clinical constructions of problems and to interrupt the oftentimes-subtle power processes that accompany and maintain them. We need to learn how clinicians maintain their resistant positions in relation to dominant discourses while working in collaborative, culturally sensitive ways (e.g., ChenFeng, Kim, Knudson-Martin, & Wu, 2017). We are now trying to discover whether SERT's discursive strategies can be identified with a coding tool and how to link this positioning work to desired client outcomes. We believe that answers require discursive-oriented practitioners study the dynamics of their work, demystifying intersections of social discourse and clinical change.

References

Baber, K. M. (2009). Postmodern feminist perspectives and families. In S. A. Lloyd, A. L. Few, & K. R. Allen (Eds.), *Handbook of feminist family studies* (pp. 56–68). Los Angeles, CA: Sage.

Bourdieu, P. (1986). The forms of capital. In J. G. Richardson (Ed.), *Handbook of theory and research for the sociology of education* (pp. 241–258). New York, NY: Greenwood Press.

Burkitt, I. (2014). *Emotions and social relations*. Thousand Oaks, CA: Sage.

Charmaz, K. (2014). *Constructing grounded theory* (2nd ed.). Thousand Oaks, CA: Sage.

ChenFeng, J. L., & Galick, A. (2015). How gender discourses hijack couple therapy-and how to avoid it. In C. Knudson-Martin, M. A. Wells, & S. K. Samman (Eds.), *Socio-emotional relationship therapy: Bridging emotion, societal context, and couples interaction* (pp. 41–52). New York, NY: Springer.

ChenFeng, J., Kim, L., Knudson-Martin, C., & Wu, Y. (2017). Application of socio-emotional relationship therapy with couples of Asian heritage:

Addressing issues of culture, gender, and power. *Family Process, 56*, 558–573. https://doi.org/10.1111/famp.12251

Collins, P. H., & Bilge, S. (2016). *Intersectionality*. Cambridge, MA: Polity Press.

Cozolinio, L. (2016). *Why therapy works: Using our minds to change our brains*. New York, NY: Norton.

Davies, B., & Harré, R. (1990). Positioning: The discursive production of selves. *Journal for the Theory of Social Behaviour, 20*(1), 43–63. https://doi.org/10.1111/j.1468-5914.1990.tb00174.x

Fairclough, N. (2016). A dialectical-relational approach to critical discourse analysis in social research. In R. Wodak & M. Meyer (Eds.), *Methods of critical discourse studies* (3rd ed., pp. 86–108). Los Angeles, CA: Sage.

Fishbane, M. D. (2013). *Loving with the brain in mind: Neurobiology & couple therapy*. New York, NY: Norton.

Foucault, M. (1973). *The order of things: An archaeology of the human sciences*. New York, NY: Vintage.

Garcia, M., Košutic, I., & McDowell, T. (2015). Peace on earth/war at home: The role of emotion regulation in social justice work. *Journal of Feminist Family Therapy, 27*, 1–20. https://doi.org/10.1080/08952833.2015.1005945

Gergen, K. J. (2006). *Therapeutic realities: Collaboration, oppression, and relational flow*. Chagrin Falls, OH: Taos Institute Publications.

Greenberg, L. S. (2007). A guide to conducting a task analysis of psychotherapeutic change. *Psychotherapy Research, 17*(1), 15–30. https://doi.org/10.1080/10503300600720390

Harré, R., Moghaddam, F. M., Cairnie, T. P., Rothbart, D., & Sabat, S. R. (2009). Recent advances in positioning theory. *Theory & Psychology, 19*(1), 5–31. https://doi.org/10.1177/0959354308101417

Hill, C. E., Thompson, B. J., & Williams, E. N. (1997). A guide to conducting consensual qualitative research. *The Counseling Psychologist, 25*, 517–572. https://doi.org/10.1177/0011000097254001

Kahn, S. A., & Monk, G. (2017). Narrative supervision as a social justice practice. *Journal of Systemic Therapies, 36*, 7–25. https://doi.org/10.1521/jsyt.2017.36.1.7

Knudson-Martin, C. (2013). Why power matters: Creating a foundation of mutual support in couple relationships. *Family Process, 52*, 5–18. https://doi.org/10.1111/famp.12011

Knudson-Martin, C. (2016). Gender in couple and family life: Toward inclusiveness and equality. In S. Kelly (Ed.), *Issues in couple and family therapy: Across socioeconomics, ethnicities, and sexualities* (pp. 153–180). New York, NY: Praeger.

Knudson-Martin, C., & Huenergardt, D. (2010). A socio-emotional approach to couple therapy: Linking social context and couple interaction. *Family Process, 49*, 369–386. https://doi.org/10.1111/j.1545-5300.2010.01328.x

Knudson-Martin, C., & Huenergardt, D. (2015). Bridging emotion, societal discourse, and couple interaction in couple therapy. In C. Knudson-Martin, M. A. Wells, & S. K. Samman (Eds.), *Socio-emotional relationship therapy: Bridging emotion, societal context, and couples interaction* (pp. 1–13). New York, NY: Springer.

Knudson-Martin, C., Huenergardt, D., Lafontant, K., Bishop, L., Schaepper, J., & Wells, M. (2015). Competencies for addressing gender and power in couple therapy: A socio-emotional approach. *Journal of Marital and Family Therapy, 41*, 205–220. https://doi.org/10.1111/jmft.12068

Krolekke, C., & Sorensen, A. S. (2006). *Gender communication theories and analysis: From silence to performance*. Los Angeles, CA: Sage.

Lobo, E., & Knudson-Martin, C. (2015). *Integrating positioning theory and neurobiology to counter gender inequality*. Roundtable. National Council on Family Relations annual meeting, Vancouver, BC, November 11.

Lorber, J. (2005). *Breaking the bowls: Degendering and feminist change*. New York, NY: W. W. Norton.

Loscocco, K., & Walzer, S. (2013). Gender and the culture of heterosexual marriage in the United States. *Journal of Family Theory & Review, 5*, 1–14. https://doi.org/10.1111/jftr.12003

McDowell, T. (2015). *Applying critical social theories to family therapy practice*. New York, NY: Springer.

McDowell, T., Knudson-Martin, C., & Bermudez, J. M. (2018). *Socioculturally attuned family therapy: Toward equitable theory and practice*. New York, NY: Routledge.

Porges, S. W. (2009). Reciprocal influences between body and brain in the perception and expression of affect. In D. Fosha, D. J. Siegel, & M. F. Solomon (Eds.), *The healing power of emotion: Affective neuroscience, development & clinical practice* (pp. 27–54). New York, NY: Norton.

Riessman, C. K. (2008). *Narrative methods for the human sciences*. Los Angeles, CA: Sage.

Samman, S. K., & Knudson-Martin, C. (2015). Relational engagement in heterosexual couple therapy: How men move from "I" to "we". In C. Knudson-Martin, M. A. Wells, & S. K. Samman (Eds.), *Socio-emotional relationship therapy: Bridging emotion, societal context, and couples interaction* (pp. 79–92). New York, NY: Springer.

Shotter, J. (2014). Methods of inquiring into "the stuff" of everyday life. In G. Simon & A. Chard (Eds.), *Systemic inquiry: Innovations in reflexive practice research* (pp. 95–123). Farnhill, UK: Everything is Connected.

Siegel, D. J. (2012). *The developing mind: How relationships and the brain interact to shape who we are* (2nd ed.). New York, NY: Guilford.

St. George, S., Wulff, D., & Strong, T. (2014). Researching interpersonal patterns. In K. Tomm, S. S. George, D. Wulff, & T. Strong (Eds.), *Patterns in interpersonal interactions: Inviting relational understandings for therapeutic change* (pp. 210–228). New York, NY: Routledge.

Strong, T. (2017). Neuroscience discourse and the collaborative therapies? In J. Duvall & M.-N. Beaudoin (Eds.), *Collaborative therapy and interpersonal neurobiology: Evolving practices* (pp. 116–127). London: Routledge.

Sutherland, O., Turner, J., & Dienhart, A. (2013). Responsive persistence. Part I: Therapist influence in postmodern practice. *Journal of Marital and Family Therapy, 39*, 470–487. https://doi.org/10.1111/j.1752-0606.2012.00333.x

Wetherell, M. (2012). *Affect and emotion: A new social science understanding.* Thousand Oaks, CA: Sage.

Williams, K. (2011). A socio-emotional relational framework for infidelity: The relational justice approach. *Family Process, 50*(4), 516–528. https://doi.org/10.1111/j.1545-5300.2011.01374.x

Williams, K., Galick, A., Knudson-Martin, C., & Huenergardt, D. (2013). Toward mutual support: A task analysis of the relational justice approach to infidelity. *Journal of Marital and Family Therapy, 39*(3), 285–298. https://doi.org/10.1111/j.1752-0606.2012.00324.x

Williams, K., & Knudson-Martin, C. (2013). Do therapists address gender and power in infidelity? A feminist analysis of the treatment literature. *Journal of Marital and Family Therapy, 39*(3), 271–284. https://doi.org/10.1111/j.1752-0606.2012.00303.x

Winslade, J. (2009). Tracing lines of flight: Implications of the work of Gilles Deleuze. *Family Process, 48*, 332–346. https://doi.org/10.1111/j.1545-5300.2009.01286.x

Wodak, R., & Meyer, M. (2016). Critical discourse studies: History, agenda, theory, and methodology. In R. Wodak & M. Meyer (Eds.), *Methods of critical discourse studies* (3rd ed., pp. 1–22). Los Angeles, CA: Sage.

8

Conversation Analysis, Discourse Analysis and Psychotherapy Research: Overview and Methodological Potential

Eleftheria Tseliou

My aim in this chapter is to discuss certain ways in which the discursive methodologies of Conversation Analysis (CA) and Discourse Analysis (DA) can methodologically add to the constantly evolving landscape of psychotherapy research, particularly concerning systemic/discursive therapies. Psychotherapy research counts decades of experimentation with a multiplicity of innovative methods for the study of how and whether psychotherapy works (for an overview, see Gelo, Pritz, & Rieken, 2015b). Correspondingly, psychotherapy process and outcome research have provided pertinent insight on the details and the effectiveness of existing variations of the talking cure. Up to date, positivist, quantitative methodological approaches have mostly offered such insight. Hermeneutic, language-based or interpretative research methodologies, known as qualitative methodologies (see Willig, 2013, for an overview), seem to occupy a marginal place in psychotherapy research, particularly as concerns outcome research (Rogers & Elliot, 2015). On the other hand, polarized

E. Tseliou (✉)
Laboratory of Psychology, Department of Early Childhood Education, University of Thessaly, Volos, Greece
e-mail: tseliou@uth.gr

O. Smoliak, T. Strong (eds.), *Therapy as Discourse*, The Language of Mental Health,
https://doi.org/10.1007/978-3-319-93067-1_8

distinctions between the "qualitative" and the "quantitative" have been questioned (e.g., Mörtl & Gelo, 2015). This has been coupled with critiques against the traditional methodological paradigm concerning its limitations to capture the complexity and the perplexity of psychotherapy (Greenberg, 2015). Such criticisms have gradually allowed space for the inclusion of a multiplicity of methodological proposals, including language-based approaches like CA and DA. CA and DA adhere to a pragmatic and action orientation approach to language. The latter implies that language use has a constitutive quality in the sense that it constructs phenomena in certain historical and socio-political contexts instead of simply mirroring them as if they were part of an independent reality "out-there" (Tseliou, 2013). Such perspective resonates with constructionist epistemology (Burr, 2015; Gergen, 1999). CA and DA have been argued as bearing potential mostly for the study of psychotherapy process, but also for the study of outcome (Elliott, 2010; Strong, Busch, & Couture, 2008) as a complementary choice to existing methodologies, as they can better address the complexity of the psychotherapeutic setting (e.g. Madill, 2015). In particular, CA and DA have been argued as bearing significant potential for the study of psychotherapy process in discursive therapies, namely, therapies espousing a systemic or constructionist theoretical and epistemological perspective (Avdi & Georgaca, 2007; Strong et al., 2008; Tseliou, 2013).

Such arguments have so far been reported in existing reviews of CA and DA studies (Avdi & Georgaca, 2007; Georgaca & Avdi, 2009; Tseliou, 2013) or in the scarce, related literature (Madill, Widdicombe, & Barkham, 2001; Madill, 2015; Pain, 2009; Spong, 2010). They mostly highlight the merit of CA and DA for the understanding of psychotherapy and report to a limited extent specific methodological aspects which may differentiate them from other existing methodologies. Consequently, the place of CA and DA in the map of psychotherapy research seems to remain relatively marginal, with limited, so far, cross-communication between psychotherapy researchers and CA/DA researchers (Avdi & Georgaca, 2007).

Instead of introducing an entirely novel line of argumentation, my aim here is to further pursue the argument concerning CA and DA potential for psychotherapy research. To do so I will focus on specific methodological aspects which I think are intrinsic to CA and to one DA trend, closely affiliated with CA, namely, Discursive Psychology (DPsy). I will argue that these aspects can potentially offer an answer to certain calls, which have been framed within a critical discussion of dichotomies like process vs. outcome or qualitative vs. quantitative.

In subsequent sections, I will start with a brief, non-exhaustive overview of the landscape of psychotherapy research in respect of the process/outcome and quantitative/qualitative divides. I will proceed with a concise account of basic CA and DA features, focusing on DPsy, as well as with a brief overview of CA and DA use in psychotherapy research. I will then explicate the main arguments concerning the methodological merit of CA and DPsy by making reference to certain notions/methodological tools and examples. Finally, I will conclude by discussing their limitations but also the implications of their deployment for the future of psychotherapy research.

Psychotherapy Research: Process and/or Outcome, Quantitative and/or Qualitative?

There are very informative, detailed historical accounts of the evolution of psychotherapy research (e.g. Braakmann, 2015; Muran, Castonguay, & Strauss, 2010). One could read these narratives in relation to two main axes. The first concerns the distinction between process and outcome psychotherapy research and the related tensions concerning its polarity. The second concerns the distinction—or similarly constructed polarity—between quantitative and qualitative methodological approaches, which extends the field of psychotherapy research.

Psychotherapy Research: From Differentiation and Polarity Towards Complementarity and Interrelation?

Psychotherapy process research, traced back to Roger's first recordings of sessions in the 1940s (Braakmann, 2015; Muran et al., 2010), is usually discussed as focusing on the study of what happens within sessions or in the process of therapy (Gelo, Salcuni, & Colli, 2012; Greenberg, 2015; Pinsof & Wynne, 2000). This focus may include research aiming to explore how an intervention works (Pachankis & Goldfried, 2007) or research aiming to unpack the mechanisms via which psychotherapy works (Hardy & Llewelyn, 2015). On the other hand, psychotherapy outcome research mostly aims at investigating the overall effectiveness of psychotherapy (Gold, 2015; Greenberg, 2015), with its historical origins placed at the decades of 1950s and 1960s (Muran et al., 2010; Pachankis & Goldfried, 2007).

As both process and outcome research aim at tackling the issue of change (how or whether it comes about), there has been extensive debate (e.g. Pinsof & Wynne, 2000) about the meaningfulness of ascribing to an ontology of the process-outcome distinction. Examples of attempts to overcome the process-outcome distinction include *change process research*, which focuses on the detailed micro-analysis of therapist and client interaction (Elliott, 2010; Greenberg, 2015) or *client-focused, progress research* (Pinsof & Wynne, 2000), where process research is defined as the study of small outcomes. Sargent (2004, p. 9) eloquently comments on the lack of meaningfulness of a strict division between process and outcome: "Since 'process' is a series of emergent outcomes, and since 'outcome' stops process at a point in time, understanding of process without reference to its outcomes is hardly conceivable".

Similarly, the prevailing, established dichotomy between quantitative and qualitative research methodologies seems gradually challenged. It is also replaced by a differentiation of approaches on the basis of epistemological preferences, like positivism/realism or relativism/hermeneutics/constructionism and on the basis of a preference for either a theory-driven (deductive) approach as opposed to a data-driven (inductive) approach.

Nevertheless, positivist research seems to dominate the field of outcome research and partly that of process research with limited use of hermeneutic, qualitative methodologies for the study of outcome (Rogers & Elliott, 2015). The latter seem deployed mostly by process studies (Hardy & Llewelyn, 2015). Outcome research seems interwoven with the logic of Evidence-Based Medicine (EBM) and the use of Randomized

Control Trials (RCTs) or a variety of experimental design types (Gold, 2015). Effectiveness is thus investigated by means of attempting to establish linear, causal relationships between models or interventions and symptom recovery, despite recent attempts to introduce non-linear perspectives along with the use of more advanced statistical models (e.g. Hayes, Laurenceau, Feldman, Strauss, & Cardaciotto, 2007; Pachankis & Goldfried, 2007; Salvatore, Tschacher, Gelo, & Koch, 2015). On the other hand, process research mostly includes various types of text analysis, where either numerical or linguistic data may be analysed semantically, that is, with the aim to identify meaning (Gelo et al., 2012). These types entail theory-driven, top-down approaches where data are checked against predefined categories or data-driven, bottom-up approaches where categories become constructed inductively (for a more extended discussion, see Gelo et al., 2012). They also include approaches investigating psychotherapy from the perspective of the researcher and his/her predefined theories as compared to participants', that is, clients' or therapist's perspective (for the latter, see, e.g., Viklund, Holmqvist, & Zetterqvist Nelson, 2010).

Psychotherapy Research and Systemic/Discursive Therapies: A Call for Conversation and Discourse Analysis Methodologies?

Both process and outcome research as well as the various methodological approaches have so far contributed to our knowledge about the psychotherapeutic endeavour in diverse and significant ways. Still, however, and particularly in the case of systemic/discursive therapies, there is need for further methodological developments of observational/naturalistic approaches, as these therapies remain under-researched especially concerning effectiveness (Heatherington, Friedlander, Diamond, Escudero, & Pinsof, 2015). As also argued elsewhere (Greenberg, 2015), both quantitative and qualitative methodologies seem to fall short of expectations to address such need for different reasons.

Systemic/discursive therapies espouse systems or constructionist theories to account both for symptom formation and change (see

Goldenberg & Goldenberg, 2008, for an overview). Instead of approaching psychotherapy process by focusing on an intrapsychic realm as concerns the "identified patient", they focus on relational, discursive patterns on the "here and now" of therapist-client dialogue. This presupposes a context-sensitive perspective which favours complexity and interdependence and prioritizes discourse, interaction and relationships as the locus for change. Quantitative approaches, like RCTs, seem unable to offer context-sensitive accounts of change on a moment-by-moment basis (Greenberg, 2015). Furthermore, effectiveness cannot be simply measured by means of the elimination of the identified patient's symptoms, given these models' interactional perspective (Friedlander, Heatherington, & Escudero, 2013). Qualitative approaches, on the other hand, forward a context-sensitive approach; however, those based on clients' narratives about sessions seemingly study what people narrate *about* psychotherapy rather than what they say or do *in* psychotherapy (Greenberg, 2015).

As a consequence, the study of change in the case of systemic/discursive therapies needs to methodologically capture the interrelatedness between client and therapist contributions (Oka & Whiting, 2013) and consequently the complexity of what should constitute the unit of analysis (Friedlander et al., 2013). This necessitates an approach with a focus on a transactional unit instead of a focus on monads, that is, the participant individuals (Knobloch-Fedders, Elkin, & Kiesler, 2015).

In the remainder of this chapter, I will argue that CA and DPsy may suggest one potential answer to the call for observational, naturalistic, context-sensitive methods, which can allow the study of systemic/discursive therapies from a change process, interactional perspective. This perspective implicates the study of change by means of a data-driven, participant rather than researcher oriented, methodological approach which locates analysis in the transactional, discursive space of the detailed moment-by-moment interaction between client and therapist. To explicate my argument, I will first briefly introduce such approaches and their up-to-date deployment in psychotherapy research. Then, I will elaborate on their specific methodological aspects which I think attend to the aforementioned call.

Conversation Analysis, Discourse Analysis and Psychotherapy Research

There are many informative accounts of CA and DA which narrate their historical evolution, the various trends and their differences (Potter, 2012; Willig, 2013; Wooffitt, 2005) as well as the details of how to approach analysis (e.g. Wooffitt, 2005). Furthermore, I have also presented these methodologies elsewhere (Tseliou, 2013, 2015, 2017; Tseliou & Borcsa, 2018). For the purposes of this text, I will briefly reiterate some key points.

Conversation Analysis

CA was founded in the 1960s by the sociologist Harvey Sacks and offers a systematic way to study how social processes are constructed by means of patterned, sequenced conversational exchanges (Sacks, Schegloff, & Jefferson, 1974). This conversational order exemplifies how meanings, social actions and identities are interactionally and conversationally constituted (Muntigl, Knight, Horvath, & Watkins, 2012). As Madill states, CA constitutes a "rigorous approach to discovering the ways in which talk-in-interaction is choreographed" (2015, p. 502). The main premise is that the social world is jointly accomplished by means of talk on a turn-by-turn basis and this process exhibits ordinariness (Atkinson & Heritage, 1984; Sacks et al., 1974; Schegloff, 2007). Speakers collaborate for the construction of meaning (Muntigl & Horvath, 2014), whereas every time that a speaker breaches order, he/she becomes accountable for this breach (Voutilainen, Peräkylä, & Ruusuvuori, 2011), like in the case where a refusal follows a request. CA research studies both everyday and institutional talk, a variation of everyday talk, where conversational practices are subject to institutional aims (Madill, 2015; Voutilainen et al., 2011). CA implies an inductive process where data are examined for patterns, which may then be examined in relation to existing theory (Madill, 2015; Voutilainen et al., 2011). Usually an initial conversational phenomenon is identified and a gradual collection of its instances follows, which are then compared and contrasted (Madill, 2015).

CA may be seen as epistemologically closer to the natural sciences paradigm as it aims for the discovery of conversational structures or rules and hence at theory building (Madill, 2015). However, following its adherence to the importance of context for the construction of meaning, CA has been argued as also ascribing to a relativist/constructionist epistemology (Rapley, 2012).

Discourse Analysis and Discursive Psychology

DA entails a multiplicity of approaches broadly espousing a constructionist epistemology (Tseliou, 2013, 2015). These either focus on the micro-analysis of language use (bottom-up) or aim to shed light to the oppressing or restraining aspects of discourse (top-down), following a post-structural discourse theory mostly inspired by the work of Foucault (1969/1972) (see Willig, 2013). There are also proposals for a both/and perspective (Wetherell, 1998). Due to my focus on DPsy here, I will not discuss top-down, DA approaches (Parker, 2015; Willig, 2013).

DPsy is considered a bottom-up approach for its close affiliation with CA, the ethnomethodological (Garfinkel, 1967) and the pragmatic, linguistic tradition of Austin and Wittgenstein, which investigates language in its use and in relation to the immediate context of such use (Lepper, 2015). It was developed as an alternative approach for the understanding of psychological phenomena, as compared to mainstream approaches in psychology. For DPsy, psychological phenomena are studied as discursive, interactional phenomena (Potter, 2012), a view similar to the one of systemic, pragmatic approaches to psychological matters (Tseliou, 2013). DPsy adheres to an action orientation perspective concerning language and incorporates a rhetorical and—in the case of Critical Discursive Psychology (Potter, 2012)—ideological perspective (Billig, 1996; Billig et al., 1988). According to the Discursive Action Model (DAM) (Edwards & Potter, 1992), talk is argumentative in that we argue for the reality and truth of our views. Simultaneously its organization attends to potential accusations for bias or interest on behalf of the speaker. To eschew such danger, discourse is often constructed as factual, that is, as discourse reporting facts and not prejudiced, personal opinions. This is accomplished by a variety of discursive strategies, like vivid descriptions, extreme case formulations and so on. Overall, talk is approached as being inherently dilemmatic and entangled with wider ideological tensions like the dilemma between rationalism and prejudice in the case of talk about national others (Billig et al., 1988).

Both CA and DPsy ascribe to an inductive perspective and retain an emphasis on the detailed, turn-by-turn, micro-analysis of discourse. In fact, DPsy has seemingly incorporated certain CA methodological contributions and utilizes the existing body of knowledge from CA empirical research to the extent that it gradually turns into CA (Potter, 2012). Yet DPsy differs from CA in that it follows a constructionist orientation while also undertaking an explicit orientation to psychological matters as compared to the mostly linguistic orientation of CA.

Overall, CA and DPsy are observational, naturalistic methods due to their preference for naturally occurring data, namely, talk and conversation as these unfold in the natural setting of their production, like transcribed audio or videotaped psychotherapeutic sessions. CA in particular, but also DPsy in most cases, further allows for the study of non-verbal aspects of talk due to the detailed transcription of its prosodic and paralinguistic features.

CA, DA and DPsy Studies in Psychotherapy Research: A Brief Overview

The use of CA and DA in psychotherapy research is not a new endeavour. CA and DA have been deployed for decades, dating back to the use of innovative language-based methodologies by Bateson among others (Peräkylä, Antaki, Vehviläinen, & Leudar, 2008a; Tseliou, 2013). Up to date, CA and DA have been used to investigate different therapy models including psychodynamic (Peräkylä, 2008), cognitive constructivist (Voutilainen et al., 2011), experiential (Sutherland, Peräkylä, & Elliott, 2014) and, mostly, systemic/constructionist (Kogan & Gale, 1997; Diorinou & Tseliou, 2014; Patrika & Tseliou, 2016; Stancombe & White, 2005; Sutherland & Strong, 2011).

Existing reviews of CA and DA studies of psychotherapy present an informative overview of "what is there" concerning the use of such methodologies by existing studies, although the field is constantly growing (e.g. Patrika & Tseliou, 2016; Sametband & Strong, 2017; Sutherland et al., 2014; Weiste & Peräkylä, 2014). Up to date there is one review aiming to highlight the contribution of DA for understanding therapy process (Avdi & Georgaca, 2007), one presenting the contribution of discursive (CA, DA) and narrative methods to psychotherapy evaluation (Georgaca & Avdi, 2009) and one systematic review investigating the methodological merit of CA and DA family therapy studies (Tseliou, 2013). Furthermore, there is limited discussion of CA potential for psychotherapy research (Madill, 2015; Madill et al., 2001; Pain, 2009; Peräkylä et al., 2008a) and of DA benefits for counsellors and counselling by a non-systematic review (Spong, 2010).

Depending on the focus of each review, CA and DA studies are clustered in groups in different ways. For example, DA psychotherapy process studies are grouped in relation to their focus concerning change, for example, as related to transformation of meanings or shifts in subjectivity or in respect of whether they undertake a micro-analysis perspective as compared to a critical, de-constructing perspective (Avdi & Georgaca, 2007; Georgaca & Avdi, 2009). Respectively, CA, DA and Narrative Analysis studies (Georgaca & Avdi, 2009) are grouped depending on whether they focus on clients' reports or therapists' interventions in respect of psychotherapy evaluation. Finally, CA and DA studies of family therapy are grouped in respect of methodological axes which include research question(s), epistemological perspective, data/sampling, type of analysis, knowledge claims and attendance to quality criteria and argued as varying in terms of methodological merit (Tseliou, 2013). They are reported as investigating various aspects of family therapy, like the conversational or discursive construction of therapeutic strategies, like neutrality (Stancombe & White, 2005) or the therapeutic relationship, for example, in the case of alliance or collaboration (Sutherland & Couture, 2007; Sutherland & Strong, 2011) or social acts like complaints (e.g. O'Reilly, 2005).

These reviews raise a number of arguments in favour of the use of CA and DA for the study of counselling/psychotherapy, particularly concerning systemic/constructionist therapies. First, CA and DA are argued as illuminating practice by offering ways to study language use at the "here and now" of therapeutic dialogue, on a moment-by-moment basis (Avdi & Georgaca, 2007; Tseliou, 2013), while investigating therapy as a "collaborative, semiotic process of meaning-making" (Avdi & Georgaca, 2007, p. 171). Furthermore, CA and DA are discussed as contributing towards bridging the gap between researchers and clinicians by enhancing therapist reflexivity, as they can highlight the effect of therapist's interventions but also issues pertaining to therapist authority and power (Avdi & Georgaca, 2007; Georgaca & Avdi, 2009; Spong, 2010; Tseliou, 2013). Finally, CA and DA approaches like DPsy are argued as facilitating the examination of how participants themselves accomplish certain conversational/relational tasks (Madill, 2015). Nevertheless, certain claimed merits are not intrinsic to CA and DA methodologies. CA and DA seem in tune with the change process paradigm in psychotherapy research (Madill, 2015). Within the latter, change is studied on a moment-by-moment basis at the micro-level of therapist and client interaction (Elliott, 2010; Greenberg, 2015) by other various types of sequential process research. As noted (Elliott, 2010), however, sequential research still seems predominated by quantitative approaches with minimal use of CA methods.

Previous reviews have contributed an indicative overview of CA and DA potential for the study of psychotherapy, thus hinting to their methodological promise. While pursuing this line of argumentation, I will focus on two interrelated methodological features which pertain to CA and DPsy. These features differentiate CA and DPsy from other methodological proposals and seem to address the need for methodological developments in psychotherapy research particularly suitable for the study of systemic/discursive therapies.

Methodological Potential of CA/DPsy for Psychotherapy Research: What Do CA and DPsy Add to Psychotherapy Research?

There are two uniquely combined features, common in CA and DPsy, which I think differentiate them from other language-based approaches in psychotherapy research. CA and DPsy bear the methodological potential for the study of change process by locating analysis within *in situ interdependent* sequences which are studied from *participants' perspective* without resorting to post-session reports or narrations about therapy. These two methodological features lead to the study of change from an interactional perspective and to the study of psychotherapy process from an "insider's view." Subsequently, I will address each in turn by explicating CA and DPsy related notions/methodological tools.

Interdependent Sequences as the Locus of Analysis: An Interactional Perspective on the Study of Change

CA and DPsy informed analysis selects interdependent sequences as the locus of analysis. There are specific CA theoretical and methodological notions, also deployed by DPsy, which are empirically grounded and make such orientation possible. These include the notions of the sequential organization of talk by means of *turn-taking*, of *adjacency pair*, of *preference structure* and *accountability*.

According to Peräkylä et al. (2008a), CA allows the examination of how social actions are sequentially constituted in talk. Turn-taking refers to the sequential organization of talk, that is, the taking of turns between speakers in conversations, subject to normative rules (Sacks et al., 1974; Schegloff, 2007; see also Madill, 2015, for examples of analysis which explicate the notions of turn-taking and adjacency pair). A series of turns, constituting a coherent whole, is a sequence.

Adjacency pairs are two turns constituting a pair, for example, question-answer, considered as the founding blocks of sequences and of social actions (Sacks et al., 1974; Madill, 2015). These actions are performed in talk and in that sense, social order is indexical (Rapley, 2012). According to Peräkylä et al. (2008a, p. 14) "adjacency pairs are the basic unit of talk." When the first part of an adjacency pair is uttered, the second is normatively expected (Sacks et al., 1974; Schegloff, 2007). A significant related notion is that of preference structure organization (Schegloff, 2007). Preference concerns the degree in which the performed action can create relational difficulties: given the structure of adjacency pairs, there are preferred and dis-preferred turns, for example, acceptance is the preferred response, following an invitation (Madill, 2015). This normative organization of talk implicates patterned regularities and indicates that while in talk-in-interaction we are socially accountable for our reports and the versions of the world and of the objects we construct. If a dis-preferred turn is uttered, then the speaker is held accountable (Schegloff, 2007). Accountability is a key notion for the DAM (Edwards & Potter, 1992), where descriptions are analytically examined in relation to the accountability concerning the reported actions but also in relation to the very choice of making the particular report. For example, if a father reports his daughter's disobedience then accountability is analytically pursued on two levels: the daughter's disobedience (content of report) but also father's choice to report it (act of reporting).

The notions of turn-taking, adjacency pair, sequential organization of talk and accountability implicate a perspective of *interdependence* and a *relational focus* as concerns turns and speakers' utterances: what is uttered is dependent upon and depends on what is previously and subsequently uttered by socially accountable speakers. Like with the systemic notion of pattern (Bateson, 1979) what is important here is not a single utterance but the way each utterance contributes to the construction of the transactional pattern in which it is embedded or else to the construction of the social action jointly accomplished by speakers. CA and DPsy analysis aims at the identification of such patterns and, most importantly, entails the methodological tools for their identification.

Participants' Perspective: The Ethnomethodological Input

This interactional analytic perspective of CA and DPsy is uniquely combined with the study of therapeutic dialogue from the perspective of participants, that is, therapist and clients, theorized in ethnomethodological terms. For ethnomethodology (Garfinkel, 1967), while in talk we constantly interpret each other's discursive contributions. Talk entails a reflexive quality, that is, reflexive markers which indicate how speakers themselves have interpreted each other's contributions in dialogue (Bozatzis, 2014). Thus, if closely examined, talk is revealing of such interpretations. This is interrelated with the notion of preference, explicated in the previous section and differentiates CA from any other kind of sequential analysis (Madill et al., 2001).

Thus, CA and DPsy analysis is grounded on how participants themselves make sense of their dialogues. Accordingly, any analytic claim concerning an action performed, that is, the construction of a blaming sequence, needs to be grounded on *participants' orientation*. The analyst needs to indicate those markers in participants' talk which exhibit the organization of a blaming sequence rather than impose such an interpretation upon data (Wooffitt, 2005). Thus the analyst needs to proceed with a careful examination of the claimed action's sequential organization as exhibited on a turn-by-turn basis, following the principles of preference organization. Each turn will indicate how the speaker has interpreted the previous turn, a principle known as "next turn proof" in CA analysis (Sacks et al., 1974, p. 729).

Furthermore, the analyst needs to examine the categories that participants themselves seem to make relevant in their talk exhibiting their own orientation. For example, the relevance of the category of the "patient" needs to be grounded on participants' talk rather than introduced by the analyst. This means that the analyst needs to look for either an explicit use of this category by participants or for descriptions which point to "category bound" activities, that is, activities interwoven with the category of a patient, like the reporting of symptoms. This analytic stance is widely known as "ethnomethodological indifference" and refers to the study of talk from an endogenous perspective, which attempts to ground analytic claims on participants' own, interactional, conversational practices as opposed to imposing the analyst's theoretical presuppositions on data (Bozatzis, 2014; Rapley, 2012).

Examples and Implications

There are many examples of CA and DPsy analysis of therapy, which explicate in detail and in practice the use of the theoretical notions I have discussed in the previous section (for CA analysis, see, e.g. Madill et al., 2001; Peräkylä, Antaki, Vehviläinen, & Leudar, 2008b; Sutherland et al., 2014; for DPsy analysis, see Diorinou & Tseliou, 2014; O'Reilly, 2005, 2007; Patrika & Tseliou, 2016; Stancombe & White, 2005). Here, I will briefly refer to two of these studies (Diorinou & Tseliou, 2014; Patrika & Tseliou, 2016) which both deployed DPsy to investigate problem talk at initial systemic family therapy sessions. In the first study, a DPsy analysis enabled the investigation of how circular questioning, the well-known systemic mode of questioning, was deployed by the therapist and responded to by family members. Analysis highlighted how circular questions seemed embedded within interdependent sequences, transformative of meaning, which seemingly forwarded a more systemic, circular perspective in problem talk (Diorinou & Tseliou, 2014). On the contrary, in the second study, analysis highlighted how circular questions seemed entangled within blaming sequences. A family member's blaming of the identified patient for the reported problem following a therapist's circular question seemed to facilitate the management of accountability issues raised in problem talk concerning family members' responsibility for the reported difficulties (Patrika & Tseliou, 2016). In both cases, analysis was performed at an interactional level and not at the level of either the therapist or the clients' contributions. Thus, for example, certain therapist questions or family members' contributions were analysed as *part of interdependent sequences*, inclusive of both therapist and family members' contributions. Furthermore, analysis was performed from an *endogenic perspective*, as markers in participants' discourse were examined in order to understand how participants themselves made sense of each other's contributions. For example, an overt denial in family members' talk as a response to the therapist's questions was analysed as indicating that the latter had been interpreted as instilling blame on family members (Patrika & Tseliou, 2016).

The use of CA and DPsy in psychotherapy research has a number of implications. First, therapist's and clients' contributions can be analytically approached as *interdependent* and as *embedded within patterned, conversational sequences*. Even in the case where the aim is to study therapist's discursive interventions, the unit of analysis remains located in *therapist and client interaction*. Secondly, theoretical notions like alliance, resistance, neutrality and so on can become translated into concrete conversational practices including the therapist's but also the client's side. Thirdly, CA, in particular, can facilitate the study of non-linguistic aspects of relational processes in therapeutic dialogue (see Weiste & Peräkylä, 2014, for an example). Fourthly, in terms of the study of process, CA and DPsy offer ways to unpack the detail of therapeutic dialogue, utterance by utterance, showing how therapist and client *interactionally/jointly* construct therapy process. This can facilitate the study of the therapeutic relationship but also—given its claimed importance for outcome (Muntigl & Horvath, 2014)—the study of change. It can illuminate how each side contributes to the process of change, how change is mutually achieved, how *therapist and client perform change together* minute by minute, utterance by utterance, and thus facilitate the *study of change in interactional processes* (Peräkylä et al., 2008a; Voutilainen et al., 2011). Given that, CA and DPsy can also add to psychotherapy outcome research in a complementary way to positivist research by shedding light to the minute-by-minute construction of outcomes (Peräkylä et al., 2008a) while studying them as conversational accomplishments (Sutherland, Sametband, Silva, Couture, & Strong, 2013). In that sense, they can facilitate the study of outcome by means of what Strong et al. (2008) define as "conversational evidence," that is, the way that client and therapist translate the therapeutic interventions into conversation and jointly accomplish psychotherapy.

Lastly, the methodological potential of CA and DPsy can more broadly forward a relational/interactional/discursive perspective of psychotherapy and of psychological phenomena, overall. This is particularly important in the case of systemic/discursive therapies which share such premises. The departure from psychological theories espoused by psychotherapeutic models, for example, concerning subjectivity, and the leaning on linguistic theories particularly by CA (Madill, 2015; Madill et al., 2001) is argued as potentially sensitizing clinicians to aspects of therapeutic dialogue which may, otherwise, remain unnoticed (Madill, 2015; Stiles, 2008). Furthermore, it can radically challenge notions like that of the autonomous subject endorsed by psychology, given the restraints posed by language/discourse (Spong, 2010).

Conclusion: Limitations and Ways Forward

I have argued that CA and DPsy bear methodological potential for the study of psychotherapy as *patterned interaction* and simultaneously *in situ* from participants' perspective. This argument reflects my own choices and preferences in my engagement with DA research, with research methodology and with systemic family therapy (for a reflexive account, see Tseliou, 2015). Furthermore it is mostly addressed to researchers rather than practitioners, despite my belief that CA and DPsy can equally constitute a source of inspiration for the latter.

CA and DPsy can alert us to obscure sides of psychotherapeutic practice (Madill, 2015) while allowing for the study of psychotherapy and change as *interactional accomplishments*. On the other hand, they "speak" a different language from the language of psychotherapy as they lean on linguistic rather than on psychological theories. This discrepancy has questioned their utility unless a mutual "translation" takes place (Stiles, 2008). Similarly, their utility is questioned concerning psychotherapeutic models which entail non-discursively theorized notions, like the psychodynamic unconscious or experience in the case of humanistic approaches. CA and DPsy cannot be considered an ideal choice for the study of change if theorized as intrapsychic, given their linguistic and pragmatic theoretical backcloth. Such issues pertain to the issue concerning the fit of a method with the theory from which it has been developed (Sargent, 2004). CA and DPsy are probably more appropriate choices for the study of models which theorize therapy and change on the level of therapist and client discursive interaction, like systemic and constructionist therapies. Nevertheless, there are voices (Heatherington et al., 2015) arguing that psychotherapy should transcend the (arbitrary) distinctions between the individual and the relational and move towards more integrative perspectives. If this were so, CA and DPsy could prove of wider utility for the study of notions, like alliance, across models.

CA and DPsy are not, of course, the "gold standard" for every kind of investigation of psychotherapy. In that sense, along with others (Elliott, 2010; Muntigl et al., 2012) I think that CA and DPsy methods are not meant to replace other traditional research methodologies but rather offer a different complementary perspective. I also think that methodological plurality is needed in psychotherapy research (Gelo, Pritz, & Rieken, 2015a), in the same sense that plurality in psychotherapy models seemingly forwards a more promising perspective for the relief of psychological distress.

So far CA and DA research has remained at a descriptive level. For example, CA research has mostly focused on the identification of conversational processes (Viklund et al., 2010) despite the fact that it could contribute to change process research due to its potential for identifying causal influences in conversational exchanges (Elliott, 2010).

Perhaps future developments will include creative cross-exchanges between CA/DPsy methods and other methods in psychotherapy research, particularly concerning CA which seems more in tune with positivist research with realist epistemological foundations. Existing examples include the case of Viklund et al. (2010) who combine CA with the significant events approach or the case of Lepper and Mergenthaler (2007) who combine CA with a quantitative type of text analysis. Another promising direction seems the use of CA for comparative designs, like in Kondratyuk and Peräkylä (2011) who compared existential with cognitive psychotherapy while studying the present moment by CA.

In any case, I think that an ongoing dialogue between CA/DA researchers and clinicians/researchers of different methodological orientations, coupled with an ongoing, critical examination of the methodological pros and cons of CA/DA could fruitfully inform the field of psychotherapy process and outcome research, as no single method can be the ideal answer to all possible queries.

References

Atkinson, M., & Heritage, J. (Eds.). (1984). *Structures of social action: Studies in conversation analysis*. Cambridge, UK: Cambridge University Press.

Avdi, E., & Georgaca, E. (2007). Discourse analysis and psychotherapy: A critical review. *European Journal of Psychotherapy and Counselling, 9*(2), 157–176. https://doi.org/10.1080/13642530701363445

Bateson, G. (1979). *Mind and nature: A necessary unity*. Glasgow, UK: Fontana/Collins.

Billig, M. (1996). *Arguing and thinking: A rhetorical approach to social psychology* (2nd ed.). Cambridge, UK: Cambridge University Press.
Billig, M., Condor, S., Edwards, D., Gane, M., Middleton, D., & Radley, A. (1988). *Ideological dilemmas: A social psychology of everyday thinking*. London: Sage.
Bozatzis, N. (2014). The discursive turn in social psychology: Four nodal debates. In N. Bozatzis & T. Dragonas (Eds.), *The discursive turn in social psychology* (pp. 25–50). Chagrin Falls, OH: Taos Institute Worldshare Books.
Braakmann, D. (2015). Historical paths in psychotherapy research. In O. C. Gelo, A. Pritz, & B. Rieken (Eds.), *Psychotherapy research: Foundations, process and outcome* (pp. 39–65). New York, NY: Springer.
Burr, V. (2015). *Social constructionism* (3rd ed.). London: Routledge.
Diorinou, M., & Tseliou, E. (2014). Studying circular questioning '*in situ*': Discourse analysis of a first systemic family therapy session. *Journal of Marital and Family Therapy, 40*(1), 106–121. https://doi.org/10.1111/jmft.12005
Edwards, D., & Potter, J. (1992). *Discursive psychology*. London: Sage.
Elliott, R. (2010). Psychotherapy change process research: Realizing the promise. *Psychotherapy Research, 20*(2), 123–135. https://doi.org/10.1080/10503300903470743
Foucault, M. (1972). *The archaeology of knowledge* (A. M. Sheridan, Trans.). London: Tavistock (Original work published 1969).
Friedlander, M. L., Heatherington, L., & Escudero, V. (2013). Research based change mechanisms: Advances in process research. In T. L. Sexton & J. Lebow (Eds.), *Handbook of family therapy* (4th ed.). New York, NY: Routledge.
Garfinkel, H. (1967). *Studies in ethnomethodology*. Englewood Cliffs, NJ: Prentice Hall.
Gelo, O. C., Pritz, A., & Rieken, B. (2015a). Introduction. In O. C. Gelo, A. Pritz, & B. Rieken (Eds.), *Psychotherapy research: Foundations, process and outcome* (pp. 1–9). New York, NY: Springer. https://doi.org/10.1007/978-3-7091-1382-0_27
Gelo, O. C., Pritz, A., & Rieken, B. (2015b). *Psychotherapy research: Foundations, process and outcome*. New York, NY: Springer. https://doi.org/10.1007/978-3-7091-1382-0_27
Gelo, O. C. G., Salcuni, S., & Colli, A. (2012). Text analysis within quantitative and qualitative psychotherapy process research: An introduction to special issue. *Research in Psychotherapy: Psychopathology, Process and Outcome, 15*(2), 45–53.
Georgaca, E., & Avdi, E. (2009). Evaluating the talking cure: The contribution of narrative, discourse, and conversation analysis to psychotherapy assess-

ment. *Qualitative Research in Psychology, 6*(3), 233–247. https://doi.org/10.1080/14780880802146896
Gergen, K. (1999). *An invitation to social construction.* London: Sage.
Gold, C. (2015). Quantitative psychotherapy outcome research: Methodological issues. In O. C. Gelo, A. Pritz, & B. Rieken (Eds.), *Psychotherapy research: Foundations, process and outcome* (pp. 538–558). New York, NY: Springer. https://doi.org/10.1007/978-3-7091-1382-0_27
Goldenberg, I., & Goldenberg, H. (2008). *Family therapy: An overview* (7th ed.). Belmont, CA: Thomson, Brooks/Cole.
Greenberg, L. (2015). Research on the process of change (1991). Commentary: Studying what people actually do in sessions: "Dream no small dreams for they have no power to move the hearts of men" (Goethe). In M. B. Strauss, J. P. Barber, & L. G. Castonguay (Eds.), *Visions in psychotherapy research and practice: Reflections from presidents of the society for psychotherapy research* (pp. 11–26). New York, NY: Routledge.
Hardy, G. E., & Llewelyn, S. (2015). Introduction to psychotherapy process research. In O. C. Gelo, A. Pritz, & B. Rieken (Eds.), *Psychotherapy research: Foundations, process and outcome* (pp. 183–194). New York, NY: Springer.
Hayes, A. M., Laurenceau, J. P., Feldman, G., Strauss, J. L., & Cardaciotto, L. (2007). Change is not always linear: The study of nonlinear and discontinuous patterns of change in psychotherapy. *Clinical Psychology Review, 27*(6), 715–723. https://doi.org/10.1016/j.cpr.2007.01.008
Heatherington, L., Friedlander, M. L., Diamond, G. M., Escudero, V., & Pinsof, W. M. (2015). 25 years of systemic therapies research: Progress and promise. *Psychotherapy Research, 25*(3), 348–364. https://doi.org/10.1080/10503307.2014.983208
Knobloch-Fedders, L. M., Elkin, I., & Kiesler, D. J. (2015). Looking back, looking forward: A historical reflection on psychotherapy process research. *Psychotherapy Research, 25*(4), 383–395. https://doi.org/10.1080/10503307.2014.906764
Kogan, S. M., & Gale, J. E. (1997). Decentering therapy: Textual analysis of a narrative therapy session. *Family Process, 36*, 101–126. https://doi.org/10.1111/j.1545-5300.1997.00101.x
Kondratyuk, N., & Peräkylä, A. (2011). Therapeutic work with the present moment: A comparative conversation analysis of existential and cognitive therapies. *Psychotherapy Research, 21*(3), 316–330. https://doi.org/10.1080/10503307.2011.570934
Lepper, G. (2015). A pragmatic approach to the study of therapeutic interaction: Toward an observational science of psychotherapy process. In O. C.

Gelo, A. Pritz, & B. Rieken (Eds.), *Psychotherapy research: Foundations, process and outcome* (pp. 515–534). New York, NY: Springer.
Lepper, G., & Mergenthaler, E. (2007). Therapeutic collaboration: How does it work? *Psychotherapy Research, 17*(5), 576–587. https://doi.org/10.1080/10503300500091587
Madill, A. (2015). Conversation analysis and psychotherapy process research. In O. C. Gelo, A. Pritz, & B. Rieken (Eds.), *Psychotherapy research: Foundations, process and outcome* (pp. 501–514). New York, NY: Springer.
Madill, A., Widdicombe, S., & Barkham, M. (2001). The potential of conversation analysis for psychotherapy research. *The Counseling Psychologist, 29*(3), 413–434. https://doi.org/10.1177/0011000001293006
Mörtl, K., & Gelo, O. C. (2015). Qualitative methods in psychotherapy process research. In O. C. Gelo, A. Pritz, & B. Rieken (Eds.), *Psychotherapy research: Foundations, process and outcome* (pp. 381–428). New York, NY: Springer. https://doi.org/10.1007/978-3-7091-1382-0_27
Muntigl, P., & Horvath, A. O. (2014). The therapeutic relationship in action: How therapists and clients co-manage relational disaffiliation. *Psychotherapy Research, 24*(3), 327–345. https://doi.org/10.1080/10503307.2013.807525
Muntigl, P., Knight, N., Horvath, A. O., & Watkins, A. (2012). Client attitudinal stance and therapist-client affiliation: A view from grammar and social interaction. *Research in Psychotherapy: Psychopathology, Process and Outcome, 15*(2), 117–130. https://doi.org/10.7411/RP.2012.012
Muran, J. C., Castonguay, L. G., & Strauss, B. (2010). A brief introduction to psychotherapy research. In L. G. Castonguay, J. C. Muran, L. Angus, J. A. Hayes, N. Ladany, & T. Anderson (Eds.), *Bringing psychotherapy research to life: Understanding change through the work of leading clinical researchers* (pp. 3–13). Washington, DC: APA.
Oka, M., & Whiting, J. (2013). Bridging the clinician/researcher gap with systemic research: The case for process research, dyadic, and sequential analysis. *Journal of Marital and Family Therapy, 39*(1), 17–27. https://doi.org/10.1111/j.1752-0606.2012.00339
O'Reilly, M. (2005). The complaining client and the troubled therapist: A discursive investigation of family therapy. *Journal of Family Therapy, 27*, 370–391. https://doi.org/10.1111/j.1467-6427.2005.0328.x
O'Reilly, M. (2007). Who's a naughty boy then? Accountability, family therapy, and the "naughty" child. *The Family Journal: Counseling and Therapy for Couples and Families, 15*(3), 234–243. https://doi.org/10.1177/1066480707301316
Pachankis, J. E., & Goldfried, M. R. (2007). On the next generation of process research. *Clinical Psychology Review, 27*(6), 760–768. https://doi.org/10.1016/j.cpr.2007.01.009

Pain, J. (2009). *Not just talking: Conversation analysis, Harvey Sack's gift to therapy*. London: Karnac.
Parker, I. (Ed.). (2015). *Critical discursive psychology* (2nd ed.). London: Palgrave Macmillan.
Patrika, P., & Tseliou, E. (2016). Blame, responsibility and systemic neutrality: A discourse analysis methodology to the study of family therapy problem talk. *Journal of Family Therapy, 38*(4), 467–490. https://doi.org/10.1111/1467-6427.12076
Peräkylä, A. (2008). Conversation analysis and psychoanalysis: Interpretation, affect and intersubjectivity. In A. Peräkylä, C. Antaki, S. Vehviläinen, & I. Leudar (Eds.), *Conversation analysis and psychotherapy* (pp. 100–120). Cambridge, UK: Cambridge University Press.
Peräkylä, A., Antaki, C., Vehviläinen, S., & Leudar, I. (2008a). Analysing psychotherapy in practice. In A. Peräkylä, C. Antaki, S. Vehviläinen, & I. Leudar (Eds.), *Conversation analysis and psychotherapy* (pp. 5–25). Cambridge, UK: Cambridge University Press.
Peräkylä, A., Antaki, C., Vehviläinen, S., & Leudar, I. (Eds.). (2008b). *Conversation analysis and psychotherapy*. Cambridge, UK: Cambridge University Press.
Pinsof, W. M., & Wynne, L. C. (2000). Toward progress research: Closing the gap between family therapy practice and research. *Journal of Marital and Family Therapy, 26*(1), 1–8. https://doi.org/10.1111/j.1752-0606.2000.tb00270
Potter, J. (2012). Discourse analysis and discursive psychology. In H. Cooper (Ed-in-Chief), *APA handbook of research methods in psychology: Vol. 2. Research designs* (pp. 119–138). Washington, DC: APA.
Rapley, M. (2012). Ethnomethodology/Conversation analysis. In D. Harper & A. R. Thompson (Eds.), *Qualitative research methods in mental health and psychotherapy: A guide for students and practitioners* (pp. 177–192). Chichester, West Sussex, UK: Wiley.
Rogers, B., & Elliot, R. (2015). Qualitative methods in psychotherapy: Outcome research. In O. C. Gelo, A. Pritz, & B. Rieken (Eds.), *Psychotherapy research: Foundations, process and outcome* (pp. 559–578). New York, NY: Springer.
Sacks, H., Schegloff, E. A., & Jefferson, G. (1974). A simplest systematics for the organization of turn-taking for conversation. *Language, 50*, 696–735. https://doi.org/10.2307/412243
Salvatore, S., Tschacher, W., Gelo, O. C. G., & Koch, S. C. (2015). Editorial: Dynamic systems theory and embodiment in psychotherapy research. A new

look at process and outcome. *Frontiers in Psychology, 6*, 914. https://doi.org/10.3389/fpsyg.2015.00914

Sametband, I., & Strong, T. (2017). Immigrant family members negotiating preferred cultural identities in family therapy conversations: A discursive analysis. *Journal of Family Therapy*. Advance online publication. https://doi.org/10.1111/1467-6427.1216

Sargent, H. D. (2004). Intrapsychic change: Methodological problems in psychotherapy research. *Psychiatry, 67*(1), 2–18. https://doi.org/10.1521/psyc.67.1.2.31253

Schegloff, E. (2007). *Sequence organization in interaction. A primer in conversation analysis I.* Cambridge, UK: Cambridge University Press.

Spong, S. (2010). Discourse analysis: Rich pickings for counsellors and therapists. *Counselling and Psychotherapy Research, 10*(1), 67–74. https://doi.org/10.1080/14733140903177052

Stancombe, J., & White, S. (2005). Cause and responsibility: Towards an interactional understanding of blaming and 'neutrality' in family therapy. *Journal of Family Therapy, 27*, 330–351. https://doi.org/10.1111/j.1467-6427.2005.00326.x

Stiles, W. B. (2008). Foreword: Filling the gaps. In A. Peräkylä, C. Antaki, S. Vehviläinen, & I. Leudar (Eds.), *Conversation analysis and psychotherapy* (pp. 1–4). Cambridge, UK: Cambridge University Press.

Strong, T., Busch, R., & Couture, S. (2008). Conversational evidence in therapeutic dialogue. *Journal of Marital and Family Therapy, 34*(3), 388–405. https://doi.org/10.1111/j.1752-0606.2008.00079.x

Sutherland, O., & Couture, S. J. (2007). The discursive performance of the alliance in family therapy: A conversation analytic perspective. *Australian and New Zealand Journal of Family Therapy, 28*(4), 210–217. https://doi.org/10.1111/j.1752-0606.2008.00079.x

Sutherland, O., Peräkylä, A., & Elliott, R. (2014). Conversation analysis of the two-chair self-soothing task in emotion-focused therapy. *Psychotherapy Research, 24*(6), 738–751. https://doi.org/10.1080/10503307.2014.885146

Sutherland, O. A., Sametband, I., Silva, J. G., Couture, S. J., & Strong, T. (2013). Conversational perspective of therapeutic outcomes: The importance of preference in the development of discourse. *Counselling and Psychotherapy Research, 13*(3), 220–226.

Sutherland, O., & Strong, T. (2011). Therapeutic collaboration: A conversation analysis of constructionist therapy. *Journal of Family Therapy, 33*, 256–278. https://doi.org/10.1111/j.1467-6427.2010.00500.x

Tseliou, E. (2013). A critical methodological review of discourse and conversation analysis studies of family therapy. *Family Process, 52*(4), 653–672. https://doi.org/10.1111/famp.12043

Tseliou, E. (2015). Discourse analysis and educational research: Challenge and promise. In T. Dragonas, K. Gergen, S. McNamee, & E. Tseliou (Eds.), *Education as social construction: Contributions in theory, research and practice* (pp. 263–282). Chagrin Falls, OH: Taos Institute Worldshare Books Publications Retrieved from http://www.taosinstitute.net/education-as-social-construction

Tseliou, E. (2017). Conversation and discourse analysis for couple and family therapy. In J. Lebow, A. Champers, & D. C. Breunlin (Eds.), *Encyclopedia of couple and family therapy*. Springer. Advance online publication. https://doi.org/10.1007/978-3-319-15877-8_941-1

Tseliou, E., & Borcsa, M. (2018). Discursive methodologies for couple and family therapy research: Editorial to special section. *Journal of Marital and Family Therapy*. Advance online publication. https://doi.org/10.1111/jmft12308

Viklund, E., Holmqvist, R., & Zetterqvist Nelson, K. (2010). Client-identified important events in psychotherapy: Interactional structures and practices. *Psychotherapy Research, 20*(2), 151–164. https://doi.org/10.1080/10503300903170939

Voutilainen, L., Peräkylä, A., & Ruusuvuori, J. (2011). Therapeutic change in interaction: Conversation analysis of a transforming sequence. *Psychotherapy Research, 21*(3), 348–365. https://doi.org/10.1080/10503307.2011.573509

Weiste, E., & Peräkylä, A. (2014). Prosody and empathic communication in psychotherapy interaction. *Psychotherapy Research, 24*(6), 687–701. https://doi.org/10.1080/10503307.2013.879619

Wetherell, M. (1998). Positioning and interpretative repertoires: Conversation analysis and post-structuralism in dialogue. *Discourse & Society, 9*, 387–412. https://doi.org/10.1177/0957926598009003005

Willig, C. (2013). *Introducing qualitative research in psychology* (3rd ed.). Berkshire, UK: McGraw-Hill.

Wooffitt, R. (2005). *Conversation analysis and discourse analysis: A comparative and critical introduction*. London: Sage.

9

Discursive Ethics in Therapeutic Encounters

Olga Smoliak, Tom Strong, and Robert Elliott

An ethos of dialogue and collaboration entered therapy in the late 1980s, mainly through how discursive or postmodern therapists challenged prevailing hierarchical and instrumental ways of practice (e.g., Anderson, 1997; Freedman & Combs, 1996; McNamee & Gergen, 1992). For discursive therapists, to practice ethically is to practice collaboratively. Seen

---

We would like to thank Eleftheria Tseliou and Peter Muntigl for their helpful comments on an earlier draft of this chapter.

O. Smoliak (✉)
Department of Family Relations and Applied Nutrition, University of Guelph, Guelph, ON, Canada
e-mail: osmoliak@uoguelph.ca

T. Strong
Educational Studies in Counselling Psychology, Werklund School of Education, University of Calgary, Calgary, AB, Canada
e-mail: strongt@ucalgary.ca

R. Elliott
University of Strathclyde, Glasgow, UK
e-mail: robert.elliott@strath.ac.uk

O. Smoliak, T. Strong (eds.), *Therapy as Discourse*, The Language of Mental Health,
https://doi.org/10.1007/978-3-319-93067-1_9

conventionally, psychotherapy is a one-way transfer of professional knowledge or influence—as interventions done *to* clients. Accordingly, meaning making in therapy tilts in favor of therapists' professional expertise and authority. In contrast, social constructionist or discursive therapists have re-conceptualized therapy as a dialogue *with* clients, based on mutual influence and privileging client expertise. While not focal in professional codes of ethics, collaboration is increasingly recognized as a guiding principle and ethical obligation of therapists (Koocher & Keith-Spiegel, 2016). Feminist, critical, and multicultural influences (e.g., Evans, Kincade, & Seem, 2011; Asnaani & Hofmann, 2012) and a growing emphasis on common factors and the therapeutic relationship (Norcross & Wampold, 2011; Wampold, 2015) have prompted this more global shift toward collaborative practice in psychotherapy.

In this chapter, we discuss, elaborate, and illustrate the ethos of collaboration ("discursive ethics," hereafter). Discursive ethics are both a distinct (discursive) perspective on professional ethics and a way of practicing therapy ethically. Our aim is to promote an awareness of therapy as discourse and explore the ethical dimension of discursively (i.e., using language) constructing meaning and action in therapy. We invite therapists, especially discursive therapists, to practice from a sensitivity to their and their clients' uses and responses to language. Our efforts to advance a discursive (or social constructionist) perspective on ethical practice are informed by our prior work (e.g., Massfeller & Strong, 2012; Strong & Busch, 2013; Strong, Busch, & Couture, 2008; Sutherland, Sametband, Gaete Silva, Couture, & Strong, 2013; Sutherland & Strong, 2011), particularly the notion of "conversational ethics" (Strong & Sutherland, 2007). We also invite therapists who do not share our constructionist premises or envision therapy as discourse to further reflect on their ways of practice, especially for the consistency between theory and how it is practiced conversationally. We begin with defining discursive ethics and outlining its underlying premises. We then present empirical illustrations of what we see as discursively ethical practice using discursive inquiry. Such analyses can offer detail and specificity by showing *how* discursively ethical practice may be accomplished interactionally. We conclude by discussing implications of our ideas and analyses for therapy practice.

Context and Definition

Ethics can be defined as "values, how we ought to behave, and what constitutes proper conduct" (Knapp, VandeCreek, & Fingerhut, 2017, p. 3). Professional ethics articulate the morality shared by members of a profession in codes of ethics that address various ethical issues (e.g., dual relationships, consent, confidentiality). Professional ethics are often seen as external to the actual processes of therapy; such processes are often framed in psychological or therapeutic, not ethical, terms (Strawbridge, 2003). Yet, therapy can be seen as an ethical (and political) endeavor, as it deals with moral judgments and promotes certain morals and norms concerning personal and relational wellbeing (Strawbridge, 2003). In other words, therapists' action and inaction have moral and political implications (Fox, Prilleltensky, & Austin, 2009; Tomm, 2003). While *content ethics* generally formulate therapists' conduct in a profession's codes of ethics, *process ethics* (Swim, St. George, & Wulff, 2001) address the process of how ethics are actualized in practice, in co-creating "ethical" and helpful therapeutic interactions. Thus, content ethics delineate how therapists *should* act to be ethical and helpful to clients, while process ethics address what therapists *actually do*, in navigating and negotiating influential and collaborative professional interactions.

For us, discursive ethics are process ethics focused on *therapy as a relational and conversational process*. In particular, discursive ethics involve a sensitivity to how both parties negotiate and shape the relations and outcomes of therapy. Discursive ethics can be examined by attending to how authority (e.g., to know, describe, explain, or determine immediate or future action) is constituted and managed interactionally and collaboratively. Discursively ethical practice should be evident in both how therapists design their descriptions of clients' experiences and proposals for action (e.g., as definitive, already determined, negotiable, requiring clients' input) and how they respond to clients' responses, including clients' disagreements and reluctance to engage in actions therapists propose. Clients can actively resist therapists' proposals and formulations (e.g., by rejecting or disconfirming) or display less active or overt resistance (Stivers, 2005). We will use the term "resistance" to refer to these client initiatives while being mindful of the term's conventional psychological connotations. We use the term the way discursive researchers use it (e.g., Ekberg & LeCouteur, 2015; Koenig, 2011; Stivers, 2005), namely, as an umbrella term that captures various kinds of actions that display or convey clients' reluctance to endorse therapists' proposals and ideas, and not as a therapeutic term that denotes clients' intrapsychic dynamics or failure to engage with professional expertise. The term "resistance" is rejected by person-centered, emotion-focused, and discursive (e.g., solution-focused) therapists on ethical grounds as unduly privileging therapist authority over client self-knowledge and agency. For us and other discursive therapists (e.g., deShazer, 1984), collaborative therapy is informed by resistance, in conversation analytic (CA) terms. In discursively ethical practice therapists seek to maximize conversational space for clients to assert their (different) understandings and preferences and treat such preferences as consequential for shaping how therapy unfolds.

Both discursive ethics and content ethics reflect the premise that therapists need to be accountable for what they do and emphasize respect for clients' knowledge, preferences, and characteristics (e.g., the American Psychological Association's [APA] Ethical Principles of Psychologists and Code of Conduct, 2017). Beyond content ethics, discursive ethics highlight therapists' sensitivities and accountability to particular clients in the immediacies of their negotiated interactions, in being accountable to their professions. Within the evidence-based practice (EBP) movement (e.g., APA, 2006) and professional codes of ethics (e.g., APA, 2017), therapists are often depicted as unilaterally handing meanings and actions over to clients (Strong et al., 2008). Common to the EBP view of practice is a one-way information transmission/reception metaphor of communication (Lakoff & Johnson, 1980) at odds with the negotiated view of professional communication underpinning discursive ethics. Our focus is instead with how meanings for clients' experiences and situations are built (articulated, implied, extended, endorsed, undermined, modified, etc.) jointly by therapists and clients in an evolving, dialogical manner. Seen through our discursive lens, "best practice" is accomplished not through therapists following a set of prescribed, empirically derived steps but through a negotiated *conversational process*: the joint construction and negotiation of meaning and coordination of action. The EBP movement and ethical codes largely overlook both (a) the conversational process of how therapists' responses are simultaneously shaped by and shaping of Heritage (1984) clients' responses in their interaction, and (b) the argumentative texture of therapy, in which meanings are negotiated and differences in understandings are worked out (or not).

Key Premises of Discursive Ethics

Discursive ethics are informed by social constructionist, discursive, and ethnomethodological perspectives in social sciences and therapy (e.g., Anderson, 1997; Billig, 1996; Edwards & Potter, 1992; Garfinkel, 1967; Heritage, 1984; McNamee & Gergen, 1992; Shotter, 1993; White & Epston, 1990). From discursive and constructionist perspectives, we have borrowed an understanding of language as constructing "reality," a focus on the micro-details of talk, and the idea that language use is political. Drawing from ethnomethodology, we see therapists and clients as active and reflexive agents focused on the interactional practices through which therapy is accomplished. Relatedly, for Garfinkel (1967), people skillfully use interpretive and interactional "procedures" or "methods" in creating and sustaining social order through culturally available procedures for making sense and co-constructing possible mutual understanding and concerted action. Thus, people are active, reflexive agents (i.e., not "cultural dopes," Garfinkel, 1967) who actively interpret situations and respond in ways that are informed, rather than determined, by cultural norms and institutional prescriptions for understanding and acting.

From an ethnomethodological perspective, people interact *accountably*, to make their meaning evident (or explicable on demand) to others with whom they interact. A speaker's description may be (dis)confirmed or (mis)understood by their conversational partner; that is, their meaning is public (rather than private) and interactionally achieved and negotiated, potentially with each speaking turn. Also significant is that people produce actions and descriptions *reflexively*, highlighting the contextual embeddedness or responsiveness of their descriptions or actions. Drawing on Garfinkel (1967), Heritage (1984) distinguished between two types of reflexivity: "the reflexivity of the actor" and "essential reflexivity" (p. 31).

While the actor's reflexivity treats actions and interpretations as the actor's individual achievement, essential reflexivity pertains to all human conduct and description in an evolving "sense" of context (activities, topics, relations, agendas, etc.), continuously redefined through responsive interaction.

Applied to psychotherapy, an ethnomethodological lens directs attention to and helps explicate practical (i.e., discursive) activities of therapists and clients through which therapy is constituted reflexively and interactionally. It presupposes that there is no therapy (e.g., clients' concerns, experiences, goals, tasks, alliance, therapeutic change, or interventions) beyond the methods therapists and clients jointly rely upon to accomplish their interaction. Clients are engaged as active contributors to and negotiators of meaning and processes, and not as passive recipients of therapists' expertise and interventions, as is often presumed within the EBP movement and ethical codes. Clients *can* and *do* exercise agency and assert their rights to know and define their experience and determine how to act in therapy—despite power differentials. They can overtly challenge and disagree with therapists' views and proposals or subtly undermine therapists' propositions and initiatives, for example, by withholding a response or minimally acknowledging therapists' offerings (e.g., Ekberg & LeCouteur, 2015; MacMartin, 2008; Massfeller & Strong, 2012; Vehviläinen, 2008). Despite being informed by broader cultural and institutional forces, we see therapy as actively negotiated by both therapists and clients.

Conceiving of clients as agents and active negotiators of therapeutic processes and meanings does not imply that how therapists act in therapy is irrelevant with respect to constraints imposed on clients or concern shown for clients' expertise and preferences. Clients in some therapeutic interactions may find it more challenging to resist therapists' offerings and to agentically contribute to a dialogue than in other interactions. What we suggest here is a variability in how therapists (or the same therapist on different occasions) work with clients. Importantly, as we have argued elsewhere (Strong & Sutherland, 2007) and are proposing here, such variability has an ethical dimension. For us, a key issue is how some therapists "dare to stay in an ongoing negotiating stance ... whereas those of other therapies are less flexible in 'sharing the floor' with clients and their preferences" (Strong, 2000, p. 145). Clearly, therapeutic dialogue does not occur by what Maturana and Varela (1988) referred to as "instructive interactionism," whereby clients robotically take up the meanings intended by therapists. The kind of ethical and reflexive dialogue that clinically and analytically interests us occurs in turn by turn conversational interactions that neither speaker can fully determine in advance, or even in the moment, however idealized the therapist's use of EBP might be. For discursive therapists (e.g., Anderson, 1997), collaborative practice is also generative practice. Therapists exclusively affirming clients' familiar understandings without offering new meanings and connections are unlikely to be transformative or therapeutic. Discursive therapists attempt to assert their expertise in ways that honor clients' expertise and preferences.

A discursive lens on ethical practice can add nuance and contextual specificity to otherwise de-contextualized, idealized, and unilaterally focused (i.e., monological) EBP accounts of practice, enabling us to capture aspects of ethical practice not captured in professional codes of conduct. In particular, it can:

- help clarify how knowledge claims are made and justified in therapy and how therapists can use expert knowledge while not compromising clients' expertise;
- offer a perspective on therapeutic interaction as messy and unpredictable rather than prescribed and "algorithmic" (Rush, 2001; Strong & Busch, 2013);
- locate therapists' actions in immediate interactional and broader sociopolitical contexts while emphasizing the reflexivity of therapists' conduct and presuming that anything therapists do (or not do) is an intervention and thus has an ethical and political dimension (Tomm, 1987);
- highlight how clients are not passive recipients of therapists' interventions but actively supply and contest meanings and courses of actions;
- treat language or discourse not primarily as a way of describing underlying experiential reality but rather as a medium of action or tool to accomplish a wide range of social and therapeutic tasks;

- explore how meanings and descriptions in therapy are multiple and negotiated, rather than presuming that there is a singular, ultimately "correct" view of clients' concerns and how to best remedy them.

Applicability of Discursive Ethics

Arguably, there is no universal, atheoretical viewpoint on how therapists should relate and interact with clients (e.g., as technical experts vs. persons in relation); "good" or "ethical" acts can only be judged with reference to a particular philosophy or understanding of moral action (Robertson, Morris, & Walter, 2007). Some therapists may not see using professional expertise collaboratively with clients as ethical practice, while others may construe and practice collaboration differently. For discursive therapists, collaboration is rooted in social constructionist and discursive perspectives of therapeutic interaction. Clearly, there is no one correct way to understand and practice therapy, and pluralism and a dialogue among proponents of different theories and philosophies are essential within the profession (Cooper & Dryden, 2016). However, therapeutic concepts and interventions can only be understood with reference to the theoretical frameworks in which they are embedded. When extracted from their underlying theories and philosophies, they can take on new meaning and prompt inconsistencies between practice and theory purportedly informing it (Safran & Messer, 1997). Collaboration thus becomes an ethical imperative for therapists who embrace social constructionist premises and understand their contributions to therapy as constructive of reality and politically consequential. For therapists adopting a realist ontology and an objectivist epistemology, collaboration is likely to be construed and practiced differently (e.g., as compliance or cooperation) than would be a therapy practiced according to social constructionist ideas.

Proponents of various approaches to therapy, such as cognitive-behavioral or emotion-focused, increasingly recognize the importance of dialogue and collaboration (e.g., Berdondini, Elliott, & Shearer, 2012; Gilbert & Leahy, 2007; Kuyken, Padesky, & Dudley, 2009). Although therapists of various theoretical orientations increasingly endorse the value of collaborating with clients, their practice often remains grounded in positivist premises, inconsistent with premises of discursive approaches informing collaboration as we have described it. Many therapists' work continues to be informed by a model of communication as unilateral transfer (from therapists to clients) of knowledge or influence (e.g., Turnbull, 2003). It also derives from the idea that clients' concerns are manifestations of deep or underlying structures and that therapists, by virtue of having specialized training and knowledge, can (and have professional responsibly to) accurately grasp and intervene upon these structures. Language, from this realist perspective, is a neutral or apolitical medium of communication and assumed to represent the reality of clients' concerns and experiences.

This is not to suggest that discursive ethics are only relevant to discursive, constructionist therapists (e.g., narrative, collaborative, solution-focused). We would argue that discursive ethics potentially extend to all therapies, as long as their practitioners enact constructionist premises in their conversations with clients. Therapists informed by constructionist ideas can use cognitive-behavioral, person-centered, emotion-focused, and other therapies (e.g., Strong, Lysack, Smoliak, & Chondros, 2019). It is thus not the question of *whether* a specific "modernist" model is used but *how* it is used. Of course, discursive and related (e.g., feminist) approaches are more consistent in their premises with a discursive perspective on ethics than other models (e.g., DSM/medical, cognitive-behavioral, psychodynamic). However, we contend any approach can potentially be used in discursively ethical ways.

Studying Ethical Practice Using Discursive Inquiry

As we argued elsewhere (Strong et al., 2008), therapy can be examined for *conversational evidence* of therapeutic change, such as changes in clients' meanings or reflections *in* therapy and in their (post-therapy) reflections *on* therapy. Conversational evidence can help widen the psychotherapy's evidence base (see Tseliou, 2018, Chap. 8), augment prevailing conceptions of evidence and methods used to evaluate therapy, and enhance helpfulness and reflexivity of therapists' practice (Strong et al., 2008). Discursive inquiry (e.g., conversation analysis or discursive psychology, both of which are informed by ethnomethodology) is well suited for generating psychotherapy's conversational evidence base, including evidence of ethical or collaborative practice. Prior discursive research has begun to identify interactional practices used to collaborate in therapy (Horvath & Muntigl, 2018, Chap. 4; Muntigl, Knight, Horvath, & Watkins, 2012; Roy-Chowdhury, 2006; Sutherland & Strong, 2011).

By examining therapy discourse in detail, we should be able to see evidence of discursively ethical practice. Discursive therapists have attempted to capture this tension with concepts of "not-knowing" (Anderson, 2005), being "decentered and influential" (White, 2007) or "directive and collaborative" (De Haene, Rober, Adriaenssens, & Verschueren, 2012). Other terms have also been used in the therapy literature more broadly, including directivity and nondirectivity (e.g., Elliott & Greenberg, 2007), treatment fidelity with flexibility (Norcross & Wampold, 2011) and responsiveness (Stiles, 2009). Although therapists carry professional authority and are sought for it, they only have secondary or indirect access to clients' "inner" experience. Clients have the ultimate epistemic (knowledge-related) authority in the domain of their experience. This may create tensions for therapists seeking to share their expertise and make proposals for therapeutic change while at the same time also not disregarding their clients' expertise and preferences (Ekberg & LeCouteur, 2015). In conversation analysis, this tension is reflected in how participants in interaction may navigate and negotiate the "epistemics of experience" and "epistemics of expertise" (Heritage, 2013).

Whereas *epistemics* deal with how participants claim, demonstrate, and contest knowledge about the world and themselves (e.g., Heritage, 2013; Potter, 1996), *deontics* denote authority to direct others' (or one's own) actions (e.g., Ekberg & LeCouteur, 2015; Stevanovic & Peräkylä, 2012). Clients may ratify therapists' deontic claims of authority, for example, by granting their proposals or may assert their deontic right to reject therapists' proposed activities. Similarly, epistemic authority may be claimed and negotiated in therapeutic interaction, as evident in therapists displaying cautiousness in interpreting clients' experience not directly accessible to them (Weiste, Voutilainen, & Peräkylä, 2016). Epistemics and deontics may be linked, or simultaneously oriented to, and managed by the participants in interaction. For example, in their analysis of cognitive-behavioral therapy, Ekberg and LeCouteur (2015) showed how clients asserted their epistemic superiority (e.g., I have already tried this and it did not work) as a way to not grant therapists' proposals for behavioral change or challenge therapists' deontic right to tell clients what to do.

The interactional management of epistemic and deontic authority in therapeutic encounters may be a way to "get at" discursive ethics. In her analysis of therapists disagreeing with clients, Weiste (2015) identified two types of disagreements: supportive and unsupportive. In supportive disagreements, therapists sought congruence between their divergent views and those of clients and "gave space" (e.g., acknowledged, sought elaboration) for clients' perspectives on their own experience. In contrast, in unsupportive disagreements, therapists discounted clients' views and challenged clients' epistemic superiority to describe and define their experience. Weiste suggested that therapists walk a fine balance in disagreeing with clients between offering potentially useful ideas and having disagreements turn into conflict that may jeopardize the positive therapeutic relationship. Similarly to Weiste, we were interested in how divergent views are produced and negotiated in therapeutic interaction in more or less ethical or collaborative ways. Discursively ethical exchanges involve sequences of actions in which therapists work at endorsing client epistemic and deontic authority and responding pro-socially (P. Muntigl, personal communication, March 16, 2018). In ethical practice, therapists offer new meanings and connections and propose activities while not compromising clients' expertise and preferences. They may:

- design descriptions of clients' experiences in ways that are grounded in clients' prior talk and that are likely to resonate for (i.e., be endorsed by) clients,
- epistemically downgrade descriptions that go beyond meanings evident in clients' prior talk,
- mitigate requests for actions and activities to which clients have not previously committed,

- redesign descriptions in face of clients' disagreeing responses to elicit firmer endorsement from clients, and
- make efforts to renegotiate constructions of clients' troubles until they are more mutually acceptable before returning to the prior activity (e.g., chair work).

These features need to be examined in their broader sequential contexts. We earlier discussed that therapists navigate a practical tension of collaborating with clients while also trying to move them out of their comfort zone and, in some cases, challenge them. Examining sequences of actions in broader contexts may show that interactions that seem less collaborative may end up being a very fruitful and overall collaborative kind of exchange. Client disagreement in itself is not a marker of non-collaboration; it may be conveying intense collaboration or opening up avenues for future collaboration.

To illustrate these interactionally accomplished features of ethical practice, we focused on sequences in which clients disagreed with therapists or denied their proposals to engage in some here-and-now action. Detailed analyses of disagreement sequences can make particularly evident the collaborative (or less collaborative) construction and negotiation of meaning and action in therapy. We used discursive psychology (DP) informed by conversation analysis (Sacks, Schegloff, & Jefferson, 1974; Sidnell & Stivers, 2013). We employed DP for illustrative purposes, rather than as a systematic way to investigate recurrent uses of particular interactional practices.

Discursive Psychology

Discursive psychology has offered sound critiques of mainstream psychology (e.g., Billig, 1996; Edwards & Potter, 1992; Potter, 1996; Tileagă & Stokoe, 2016; Wiggins, 2017). Whereas psychology and psychotherapy often adopt a cognitivist approach that envisions psychological phenomena (e.g., emotion, attribution, memory, traits, attention) as internal processes and entities, DP re-specifies these phenomena as externally observable discursive accomplishments or matters that people orient to and construct with their talk (e.g., Edwards & Potter, 1992). For example, it investigates "emotion discourse" or how people describe and invoke emotions in their everyday interaction (Edwards, 1999). DP treats psychological categories of emotion, cognition, agency, dispositions, and so forth as both *occasioned*, that is, embedded in a particular interactional context, and *rhetorical*, that is, concerned with actual or anticipated alternative descriptions. It attends first to how people evoke and reference mental states ("I am angry," "I don't know," "I thought that") and second to the interactional business performed by such terms and descriptions (e.g., blaming, defending, inviting, complimenting). For example, "I don't know" may be used to mitigate one's stake or interest in producing a particular description of events or people. Although emotional and other mental states are situationally produced, there are cultural or institutional vocabularies and prevailing meanings concerning experience that inform (and constrain) the local production and negotiation of meaning (Billig et al., 1988; Potter & Wetherell, 1987). DP is concerned with observable issues of fact and accountability (Edwards & Potter, 1992). By producing certain descriptions of events and people, speakers manage to imply certain things about themselves and others, for example, suggesting that the other person is accountable for their actions and is to blame for something (*accountability*). At the same time, by referencing, displaying, or invoking emotions, memories, or thoughts, speakers demonstrably produce descriptions as factual and disinterested, that is, minimize their stake and interest in producing these particular descriptions (*fact construction*).

Examples of Ethical Practice

Below, we present three extracts from different sessions of emotion-focused therapy (EFT), each involving a different client and the same therapist. In these examples, therapists make and justify claims to know clients' inner experience. Each example illustrates one or more features of discursively ethical practice we identified above. The examples are taken from a collection of ten recordings of EFT for social anxiety collected in Scotland (Elliott, 2013) and involving chair work, a well-known EFT intervention (e.g., Elliott, 2013; Greenberg, 2015). These data were chosen for pragmatic reasons (due to their availability) and because EFT therapists strive to balance directivity and nondirectivity (e.g., Elliott & Greenberg, 2007; Greenberg, 2014). EFT concerns the construction and negotiation of meaning, with the focus on emotions or, as DP scholars would put it, emotion discourse (Edwards, 1999). Angus and Greenberg (2011) argued, "psychotherapy is a specialized discursive activity designed to help clients shape a desired future," with the focus on "the role of reflection on emotion in the creation of meaning and identity" (pp. 3–4 and 7). We should be able to see conversational evidence of how clients and therapists construct and negotiate descriptions of clients' emotional and cognitive processes collaboratively. An appreciation of the ethical/collaborative dimension of EFT practice can be enhanced by explicating the largely taken-for-granted interactional processes of EFT. In the examples we present, therapists and clients are engaged in a two-chair dialogue involving either an imagined dialogue between a critical part of self and another part that is the object of this criticism or a dialogue between nurturing and nurtured parts of self. Clients are asked to alternate between enacting different parts of self by moving back and forth between the chairs.

In Example 1, the client does not endorse the therapist's formulation of her troubles. In response, the therapist engages in additional interactional work to renegotiate the meaning of her troubles or distress before returning to the prior activity of chair work. The participants discuss the client's fear of other people ("social anxiety") and negotiate the meanings and sources of the "dread" or anxiety she experiences in social situations. The therapist addresses the client's inner critic and inquires about how the critic evokes anxiety in the other, distressed part of the client's self. The names in transcripts are pseudonyms, and informed consent was obtained for all recordings (see Table A.1 in Appendix).

(1) SA-273, 7.25 Minutes into Session 16 (Audiorecording)

```
THP:  ... what do you do to fill her with dread?
CLI:  U:m (3.8) I suppose, (.) ju::st  (0.6) listing all those
      negatives
THP:  All those negatives >okay that< that’s enough to fill her with
      drea:d (0.4) >so let's go through it again< one more time then
      >what are the negatives< (0.4) .hh cos you do this >over and over
      again< don’t you,(0.4) run through the list over and over again?
      (0.8)
CLI:  ↑Kind of
THP:  Kind of ↑okay [not totally okay]
CLI:                [I don’t know    ] (0.4) I never really  pay
      attention to what happens it’s just a feeling of dread
      (0.6)
THP:  Ri:ght okay, (.) ↓ri:ght
      (0.4)
CLI:  And like if I think about it I get the negatives
THP:  Yeah we’re trying to we’re actually trying to:: (.) to it’s
      automated (.) it’s automatic it’s an automatic ↑process right
CLI:  Yeah
THP:  You do (.) yeah so we’re trying to actually just slow it do::wn
      (.) .hh and open it u:p and see how it wo:rks get inside of it
      and f- to do that we actually have to ena:ct it (.) he:re
CLI:  U::m (0.4) [oka:y   ]
THP:             [Cos it’s] (like) that’s how you de-automate it (.)
      does that make sense? (.) [It’s a standard ps]ychology thi::ng
      right=
CLI:                            [↑Yeah huh huh]
THP:  =Yeah .hh it’s not just in this therapy right ↑huh huh [ha ha]
CLI:                                                         [Ye:s ]
      (.)
CLI:  ↑U::m
      (.)
THP:  °So°
      (0.4)
CLI:  .tch .hh (.) so: (.) I suppose the feelings have been (.) boring,
THP:  You’re bori:ng
CLI:  Self conscious about appeara:n[ce about]
THP:                                [Aha you d]on’t look [nice] yeah
CLI:                                                     [Just]
      Socia:l  (.) skills in ge[neral ]
THP:                           [You’re] not socially skilled you put
      people o::ff
```

According to the therapy literature, the second step of the EFT two-chair work for conflict splits is Entry into Chair Work. To accomplish this step, the therapist seeks to “promote the client owning of experience” (Elliott & Greenberg, 2007, p. 247). To ask the client to enact self-criticism in the session, the client needs to endorse the notion that self-criticism is a relevant aspect of her experience. We see two competing formulations of the client's troubles: the inner critic actively produces anxiety in the client's mind and criticism and anxiety emerge unexpectedly and outside of the client awareness (i.e., their source is unknown). The therapist's initial question (line 1) embeds the presuppositions that there is a mental split with the client and that the client (as the inner critic) actively "does" something to make the other part of self feel anxious ("what do you do to fill her with dread?" line 1). The question implicitly attributes agency to the client (the inner critic in her) for her own distress and advances the institutional (EFT) perspective on the client's distress. The therapist's question (line 1) displays a preference for an agreeing response from the client that the critic creates distress in the client's mind. The therapist further presents self-criticism not as a singular occurrence but as an instance of a scripted mental pattern (Edwards, 1994) ("over and over again," also note the verb tense in "run through" and "do" which implies recurrence or routineness of actions; lines 6–7). He further formulates self-criticism as a sufficient and exhaustive cause of distress ("that's enough to fill her with drea:d"; line 4). The description of the client as predisposed to self-criticism and as actively "doing" criticism in her mind supplies a warrant to examine and enact self-criticism in therapy. The therapist's proposal ("let's go through it again," line 5) initiates the inner critic's criticizing of the other, vulnerable part of self.

The client is reluctant to endorse the therapist's formulation of her distress. In CA terms, she resists attribution of agency and the construction of her as routinely engaging in self-criticism. Although she answers the therapist's initial question and, in so doing, implicitly endorses the idea that the inner critic actively criticizes the other part of self (lines 2–3), her answer already displays reluctance and discomfort with the therapist's description of her troubles. Conversation analysts have observed that, across a variety of settings, to signal support and solidarity people avoid or minimize disagreements, disconfirmations, and rejections and maximize agreements, confirmations, and acceptances. Agreement is produced without delays and with marked enthusiasm, and disagreement is produced with silences, turn prefaces (e.g., *well, um*), partial repeats, and other markers of reluctance to agree (Pomerantz, 1984; Pomerantz & Heritage, 2013). The client's turn is designed with delay devices (turn preface *u:m* and a long pause) marking an upcoming dispreferred, disagreeing response (Pomerantz, 1984). The client omits herself as the subject enacting self-criticism ("just listing all those negatives") (Oh, 2006) and downgrades her commitment to the idea that negative self-talk is the source of her dread ("I suppose…"). Disagreement is even more evident in her subsequent response (lines 9–16), in which she asserts a partial or qualified (disagreement implicative) agreement (↑Kind of) (Pomerantz, 1984) and an account justifying her disagreeing response. The account helps mitigate her agency by presenting negative self-talk as emergent outside of her control ("if I think about it I get the negatives"; line 16). She further evokes the psychological category of "attention," specifically the claim that she is inattentive to the workings of her mind (lines 11–12), to deflect the notion that dread is of her own doing.

The client not endorsing the therapist's construction of her troubles undermines the therapeutic relevance of chair work. Rather than progressing with the therapeutic activity of chair work (e.g., reissuing the proposal that the critic criticizes the other part of self), the therapist attempts to first renegotiate the construction of the client's troubles, a sign of a discursively ethical practice. He acknowledges, rather than disregards, the client's response ("Kind of ↑okay not totally okay," line 10). Specifically, he repeats the client's response, produces the sequence closing third (okay), and then reformulates it with "not totally." "Not totally" reworks the meaning of "kind of" toward agreement as in "almost right" rather than disagreement as in "maybe not." The therapist's acknowledgement of the client's response elicits the client's overlapping elaboration of "kind of" (lines 11–16) and may be a way to get the client elaborate on her views.

While acknowledging the client's disagreeing view, the therapist does not abandon and continues to advance his views. He attempts to legitimize *his* perspective on her troubles with an account evoking his professional expertise in the domain of how human mind and therapy work (lines 17–28). The account references temporal and spatial metaphors ("slow it do::wn (.) .hh and open it u:p," "get inside of it") that keep the description of the proposed activity global and vague. Vagueness, as Potter (1996) suggests, "may provide just enough detail material to sustain some action without providing descriptive claims that can open it to undermining" (p. 118). Following the account, with "so" (line 33), the therapist elicits the client's granting of his proposal that she criticizes herself. The client fulfills the therapist's proposal to review her anxiety-provoking internal discourse but resists the activity of chair work. She lists the negative messages *to the therapist* rather than *to the other part of self* (i.e., does not engage in the two-chair dialogue). The therapist corrects her by inserting the second person pronoun "you" while leaving intact other elements of the client's turns (lines 36, 38, 41–42). Correction works to elicit the client's direct engagement with and criticism of the other part of her self.

Features of the discursive accomplishment of ethical practice we wish to highlight include the therapist offering his ideas not as definitive but as uncertain and requiring input from the client. He observably treats the client as having epistemic authority in the domain of her experience (note the tag "don't you" and a rising or questioning intonation on line 7). Her understanding of her own experience is observably relevant to the therapist, as he elicits her views (lines 1) and her endorsement of his ideas (lines 7 and 25). Formulating his requesting turn as a proposal for joint action (let *us* go through it again) is a way to share deontic authority with the client and invite collaboration from her in the decision-making concerning what happens in therapy (Ekberg & LeCouteur, 2015; Stivers et al., 2017). Finally, he makes efforts to negotiate the construction of the client's distress before returning to the prior activity.

We see additional opportunities to enhance the ethical potential of this interaction. The therapist's speaking turns (lines 4 and 17) offer opportunities to (a) attend to the client's displayed reluctance to accept his views; (b) further explore *her* perspective on her troubles, including her views on the value of understanding her distress in EFT terms or as related to the split between critical and criticized parts of her self; and (c) develop a mutually acceptable construction of the client's troubles. Possible therapist responses could include: I am noticing that what I am offering does not fully fit for you. I see the dialogue between the critical and criticized parts of self as relevant and important and your distress as rooted in this dynamic, but this understanding may not resonate for you. Could you say more about how you make sense of "dread"? What are your thoughts on my idea that dread is the product of self-criticism and my proposal to enact self-criticism in the session? Is there another way for us to address dread that may work better for you?

Example (2) illustrates similar features of ethical practice. It involves the two-chair dialogue for conflict splits and the collaborative construction and negotiation of the client's troubles (the client is different from the client in Example 1). The client is asked to enact a critical part of self and criticize the other part of self. On line 6, the therapist addresses the inner critic part of the client and requests that the critic talk to the vulnerable or experiencing part of self imagined in the empty chair.

(2) SA-276, 24.05 Minutes into Session 13 (Videorecording)

```
THP:  Okay so wha- >what is it< what is (.) what does happen
      (1.4)
CLI:  I get anxious::s like (.) I find it really difficult to make (.)
      eye contact (0.4) and I also find it difficult to like (.)
      remember things to say
THP:  Okay (0.4) .hh so make it (.) so tell her not to make eye
      conta::ct ((points to the empty chair))
CLI:  Don't make eye conta:ct
THP:  °Yeah° what >how do you< do that how do you get her not to make
      eye conta:ct (0.4) do you shame he:r?
CLI:  Jus- sort of like (.) can't make eye contact
      (0.4)
TRP:  .hh n- no:w no- ma- n- not ma:king eye contact often (.) goes
      with sha:me °right° (.) cos when you feel shame you kind of wanna
      shrink in and hide yourself and look awa:y (.) is that what you
      do do you shame [her ]
CLI:                  [Yeah] I think,
THP:  Okay so shame her ((points to the chair))
      (.)
CLI:  ↑s- (.) ↓hu:h .hhh I'm not $su:re how$ hhh
      (0.4)
THP:  You should be ashamed of yourself you're (0.4) not worthy, you're
      no::t (°liked°)
CLI:  Yeah you're not worthy you don't dese:rve (.) this,
THP:  You don't dese::rve this attention
CLI:  Yeah
THP:  You don't deserve this attention (.) why why doesn't she deserve
      this attention
      (1.8)
CLI:  Um, (.) I don't $kno(h)w$ .hhh
      (.)
THP:  °Don't kno:w° (.) okay so it's not a why:: it's just you don't
      deserve it
CLI:  Yeah
THP:  Right (0.4) (right) it's not right for you to have this (.) you
      don't deserve it (.) no you're not worthy of it (0.4) what is she
      the:n if she's not worthy of it
CLI:  She's ↑nothi:ng she's >never going to< (.) get anywhe:re or do
      anythi:ng ((starts crying))
THP:  You're nothing tell her ((points to the chair)) you're nothing
      (0.4) you're not gonna:,
CLI:  You're <nothing>
THP:  Yea:h yeah does that fit? (0.4) That's what it feels like huh (.)
      Okay (.) change ((points to the chair))
```

The therapist's polar (yes/no) question (line 10) is designed to elicit an agreeing response from the client or a confirmation that she shames or criticizes herself. On the surface, the therapist's question honors the client's epistemic superiority (the therapist is seeking an answer from the client). However, the question's yes/no format discourages the client from asserting her epistemic authority. The question advances a particular institutionally relevant hypothesis (and the therapist's epistemic authority) by constraining the client to answer with *yes* or *no*, preferably *yes* (Bolinger, 1978; Raymond, 2003). In response, the client contests the polar question's presupposition that she shames herself and the constraints imposed by its polar (yes or no) format by producing a dispreferred or nonconforming response ("Jus- sort of like (.) can't make eye contact," line 11). She answers the therapist's initial how-question ("how do you get her not to make eye conta:ct") rather than the turn-final polar question ("do you shame he:r?"). Instead of issuing *yes* or *no* or a similar response (e.g., I shame her), she reissues her prior claim of inability to make eye contact in social situations (line 11).

Similarly to Example (1), to advance his therapeutic agenda and rhetorically manage the client's reluctance to endorse his proposition that she has a propensity to self-criticize, the therapist evokes his superior professional expertise. He offers an account (lines 13–15) linking the "avoidance of eye contact" with "shame" by referencing what people in general routinely do and experience (note "often goes" in "not ma:king eye contact often (.) goes with sha:me," and the second person pronoun *you* marking an unspecified or generic other in "when you feel shame you kind of wanna shrink in and hide yourself and look awa:y"). The account is epistemically downgraded (note restarts and pauses) or offered tentatively. In response to the therapist's reissued polar question (line 17), the client produces a reluctantly performed agreement ("Yeah I think"). The two-chair activity is resumed with *So* + the imperatively formatted "shame her" (line 18). The therapist is treating the client's response as strong enough endorsement, when it was produced weakly. The therapist coaches the client to speak as the inner critic (lines 22–25) when she observably struggles to produce shaming speech. He then elicits an explanation from the client concerning reasons for the inner critic's negative perception of her (lines 27–28). After acknowledging her answer ("Don't kno:w° (.) okay"), he reverts back to the description that has been established as mutually endorsed ("so it's not a why:: it's just you don't deserve it," lines 32–33), confirmed by the client in the next turn (line 34). This is an instance of the therapist adjusting his talk in light of the client's response.

The features of ethical practice observed in Example 1 can also be noticed here. The participants negotiate a more mutually acceptable understanding of the client's trouble (lines 9–17) before resuming chair work (line 18). We also see the therapist epistemically downgrading his formulation of the client's experience (lines 13–16) and seeking information from the client concerning her inner experience (lines 1 and 36–37). In designing the critic's shaming speech, both participants orient to the client's epistemic superiority (note her confirming the content supplied by the therapist on lines 24 and 26 and the information seeking question on lines 36–37). We identified additional opportunities to collaboratively develop meaning and action in this stretch of talk. The therapist could have further explored the client's views on her troubles and reluctance to fully endorse his proposition that the inner critic shames her (lines 11 and 17) before adding legitimacy/authority to his views and resuming chair work (lines 13–18). The question that elicits the inner critic's views of the client could have been asked earlier (line 22). That way, the client could be the one to supply the content of the shaming speech (as she does on lines 37–38), rather than merely confirming and recycling the content supplied by the therapist (lines 24–34).

Example (3) shows the interactional accomplishment of another EFT task, namely, compassionate self-soothing (e.g., Goldman & Greenberg, 2013). This Example is a good illustration of the therapist asserting epistemic (and deontic) authority and the client challenging the therapist's right to describe experience and determine the client's in-session actions. Previously, the client identified "god" as someone who can show compassion to her. In this stretch of talk, the therapist addresses the client (as god) and asks god to convey compassion to the client imagined sitting in the other chair.

(3) SA-011, 42.02 Minutes into Session 8 (Videorecording)

```
CLI:  Think you're mo::re than just okay that you're, (0.4) to me that
      you're per↑fe:ct (.) as you ↑a::re,
THP:  (.) tell her how she's perfect, tell her (0.4) what's perfect
      about her
CLI:  ↑What's perfect about you i::s ↑u:::m,
THP:  °What's something else that's good about her?°
      (1.8)
CLI:  E::r
      (4.2)
THP:  °You care about other people°
CLI:  A::h you do (.) care about other people, (.) u::m and at ti::mes
      you ge::t (0.4) e:::r
THP:  What else
CLI:  You stop ya-
THP:  °(?)°
CLI:  You ca:::re you lo:::ve (0.6) you're so  ki:nd to:: (0.6) you
      just love anima::ls,
20 lines omitted
THP:  Hmm mm (.) tell her how she looks (.) °tell her how she looks°
      ((points to the chair))
      (0.4)
CLI:  U::m, (3.6) er (5.6) I don't know I don't think think god see::s
      (.) me [as I ] loo::k (.) ↑how I look I think
THP:         [O:kay]
THP:  Okay (cos) how does god see you:,
CLI:  U:::m  (2.6) I ↑think god just god sees me as a (.) u::m
      (0.4)
THP:  Sees you:r (.) beautiful sou:l
CLI:  Aye as a feeling person,
THP:  Oka::y
CLI:  (     ) (.)  ↑tha::t's what u:::m (.) how go::d, (0.4) I >don't
      think<, (0.4) go::d is
THP:  It do[esn't] matte::r (.) >°okay so< tell her (.) .hhh it=
CLI:       [Here ]
THP:  =doesn't matter how you look (.) [I accept ] you a- as you=
CLI:                                   [(It does)]
THP:  =look
CLI:  It ↑does nae ↓matter how you look, [and    ] it never ↑has=
THP:                                     [(Good)]
CLI:  done, coz I just e:r (.) I look at you (.) and your ↑mi:ne
```

The therapist issues a series of directives (lines 3–4, 19–20, and 33) aimed at getting the client (as god) to validate herself. The client, after some displayed difficulty and prompting and assistance from the therapist, complies (lines 11–12, 16–17) by listing her positive qualities. The second directive (lines 19–20) is met with non-compliance from the client (lines 22–23); the therapist directs god to convey content that does not "fit" the client. Whereas the first directive ("tell her how she's perfect," line 3) builds on the content supplied *by the client* in the prior turn ("you're perfect," line 2), in the second directive ("tell her how she looks," line 19), the content to be conveyed in the dialogue between the client and god is offered *by the therapist* (i.e., not yet shared or mutually endorsed). The client evokes her superior epistemic access to and right to explain her own experience as a way to challenge his epistemic claims and deontic authority to direct her actions in therapy. Specifically, she mobilizes the psychological category of "perception" and describes god's perception as a way to resist the therapist's agenda and justify her non-compliance with his directive.

We observe how the participants' (therapist's, clients', god's) differential epistemic authority is constituted in this interaction. Specifically, god is presented as the most knowledgeable about how "he" sees the client, the client as less knowledgeable than god but more knowledgeable than the therapist, and the therapist as the least knowledgeable. Rather than presenting her description of how god sees her as factual (e.g., god does not care about how I look), the client builds up the description as provisional by grounding it in her own reasoning ("I don't think think god see::s (.) me," "I ↑think god just god sees me as (.) u::m," "I >don't think<, (0.4) go::d is," lines 22, 26, 31–32) and claiming uncertainty ("I don't know," line 22). The client implicitly constitutes herself as someone who does not have direct access to god's mind and who is not entitled to know with certainty god's perceptions. Epistemic downgrading may be a way to mitigate or soften the refusal component of the turn.

Although the client is treated as less knowledgeable than god about god's perceptions, she is presented as more knowledgeable than the therapist, as evident in the therapist eliciting information from the client about how god sees her (line 25) and the client supplying information (line 26) and confirming the therapist's understanding ("Aye," line 29). The client claims epistemic authority in how *her* significant other (god) sees her and, in so doing, undermines the therapist's claim of deontic authority or his power to direct the client's actions in therapy and evokes her deontic right to say no to his proposed activities. In the third directive, the content the therapist asks god to convey to the client ("tell her (.) .hhh it doesn't matter how you look," lines 33–35) is a gist of the client's prior talk and is mutually endorsed by the client and therapist and, not surprisingly, we see compliance with the directive and no reluctance from the client (lines 38–40).

As in the prior Examples, the therapist's commitment to his institutional (EFT) agenda occurs alongside the therapist ethically responding to the client. He seeks and acknowledges the client's perspective and honors her reluctance to fulfilling his request and does not push god to discuss the client's appearance (lines 25, 28, 30, 33). His final directive *to tell* (line 33) builds on or incorporates the client's preferences regarding the precise content of what god would say to her. The client here is not passive and does not unquestionably follow the therapist's initiatives, but asserts her preferences and expertise in the domain of her own experience. Despite potential threats to solidarity, she issues a dispreferred, non-complying response (note delays, preface *um*, mitigating *I don't know*) (lines 22–23). The therapist does not abandon his line of intervention when faced with resistance from the client and continues facilitating the dialogue between god and the client. While the *content* of what god says is adjusted in light of the client's responses (evidence of the therapist responding in ethical ways), the institutional *activity* of the client as god validating herself is preserved (lines 3–4, 10, 13, 19, 33–35). The therapist also coaches the client is how to properly talk as god (lines 10 and 39). The therapist is also observably eager to move forward with the chair work, as evident in multiple and overlapping "okays" (lines 24, 30, 33) that work to close down the question-answer sequence that clarifies how god sees the client (lines 25–29) and begin a new (directive-response) sequence that resumes the chair work (line 33). The therapist could have further explored the client's perspective on how god sees her.

Conclusion

In this chapter, we proposed discursive ethics as an important but frequently overlooked aspect of ethical practice. We also offered preliminary evidence of discursive ethics in action: clients actively participating in therapeutic dialogues and contesting meanings and initiatives proposed by therapists and therapists evoking and using their (culturally and institutionally afforded) authority ethically. Foucault (1979) once criticized professionals for requiring docility from their clients to do their work, and this presumes a kind of professionalism with which we disagree. Discursive therapists have explored how therapists can reflexively elicit and respond to client resistance or markers of disagreement (e.g., deShazer, 1984). Consistent with these concerns, a greater focus on collaboration between therapists and clients in their conversational work has been evolving, and what we have been describing as discursive ethics fit within the recurring research conclusions that a strong "working alliance" (see Horvath & Muntigl, 2018, Chap. 4) is important to effective practice. Central to a working alliance is client-therapist agreement on the tasks of therapy, and we have been examining communicative interactions of therapy as an often-overlooked dimension of those tasks.

The ideas we discuss are not inconsistent with counseling professions' guidelines for best practice. For example, the APA Presidential Task Force on Evidence-Based Practice (APA, 2006) defined evidence-based practice as "the integration of the best available research with clinical expertise *in the context of patient characteristics, culture, and preferences*" (p. 271, emphasis added). In addition to matching interventions to clients, the Task Force urged practitioners to develop goals "in collaboration with the patient and consider the patient and his or her family's worldview and sociocultural context" (p. 276). A new dimension we introduce concerns the reflexivity of client and therapist conduct. Rather than envisioning clinical and research expertise and clients' characteristics and preferences as already "there," the discursive view we advance sees them as emergent and constituted *through* therapists' and clients' actions in their interaction. With particular questions, reflections, interpretations, and other responses, therapists offer and negotiate meanings and ways of "doing" therapy; such constituted contexts, in turn, shape therapists' and clients' subsequent actions and interaction. With their overreliance on the metaphor of communication as unilateral transfer of information between therapy participants, the APA Task Force and counseling professions more broadly overlook how therapists' talk helps bring forward particular "realities" and overlook alternatives. The process of meaning construction and negotiation can be seen as an integral part of "implementing" an empirically supported treatment, but is often overlooked in therapy research focused predominantly on therapists' behaviors seen as divorced from clients' responses and the interactional context. The concept and illustrations of discursive ethics can help therapists: (a) sensitize to how their work is discursive and interactional, (b) recognize how multiple, potentially competing descriptions and ways of working together are possible, and (c) consider ethical and political dimensions in their participation in therapy with respect to how their contributions help bring about certain (e.g., institutional) realities and ways of talking and bypass other realities, each with associated political and ethical implications.

To conclude, we note that the approach now known as EFT (but then referred to as process-experiential psychotherapy; Greenberg, Rice, & Elliott, 1993) began with the formulation of a set of six therapeutic principles, which the authors identified from their practice as therapists: empathic attunement, therapeutic bond, task collaboration, supporting emotion processing, offering growth/choice, and encouraging task completion. All of these principles can be observed in the three examples of therapeutic discourse analyzed in this chapter. At the time, Greenberg and colleagues framed these broad guidelines as similar to ethical principles. Discursive ethics, however, highlight that these principles are not *similar* to ethical principles; they *are* fundamentally ethical in nature, and are constantly played out in the moment-by-moment interaction between client and therapist.

References

American Psychological Association. (2006). Evidence-based practice in psychology. *American Psychologist, 61*(4), 271–285.

American Psychological Association. (2017). *Ethical principles of psychologists and code of conduct* (2002, Amended June 1, 2010 and January 1, 2017). Retrieved from https://www.apa.org/ethics/code/ethics-code-2017.pdf

Anderson, H. D. (1997). *Conversation, language, and possibilities: A postmodern approach to therapy*. New York, NY: Basic Books.

Anderson, H. D. (2005). Myths about 'not-knowing. *Family Process, 44*, 497–504.

Angus, L., & Greenberg, L. (2011). *Working with narrative in emotion-focused therapy: Changing stories, healing lives.* Washington, DC: American Psychological Association.

Asnaani, A., & Hofmann, S. G. (2012). Collaboration in culturally responsive therapy: Establishing a strong therapeutic alliance across cultural lines. *Journal of Clinical Psychology, 68*(2), 187–197.

Berdondini, L., Elliott, R., & Shearer, J. (2012). Collaboration in experiential therapy. *Journal of Clinical Psychology, 68*(2), 159–167.

Billig, M. (1996). *Arguing and thinking: A rhetorical approach to social psychology* (2nd ed.). New York, NY: Cambridge University Press.

Billig, M., Condor, S., Edwards, D., Gane, M., Middleton, D., & Radley, A. (1988). *Ideological dilemmas: A social psychology of everyday thinking.* London: Sage.

Bolinger, D. (1978). Yes/No questions are not alternative questions. In H. Hiz (Ed.), *Questions* (pp. 87–105). Dordrecht: Reidel.

Cooper, M., & Dryden, W. (Eds.). (2016). *The handbook of pluralistic counselling and psychotherapy.* London: Sage.

De Haene, L., Rober, P., Adriaenssens, P., & Verschueren, K. (2012). Voices of dialogue and directivity in family therapy with refugees: Evolving ideas about dialogical refugee care. *Family Process, 51*(3), 391–404.

de Shazer, S. (1984). The death of resistance. *Family Process, 23*(1), 11–21.

Edwards, D. (1994). Script formulations: A study of event descriptions in conversation. *Journal of Language and Social Psychology, 13*, 398–417.

Edwards, D. (1999). Emotion discourse. *Culture and Psychology, 5*, 271–291.

Edwards, D., & Potter, J. (1992). *Discursive psychology.* London: Sage.

Ekberg, K., & LeCouteur, A. (2015). Clients' resistance to therapists' proposals: Managing epistemic and deontic status. *Journal of Pragmatics, 90*, 12–25.

Elliott, R. (2013). Person-centered-experiential psychotherapy for anxiety difficulties: Theory, research and practice. *Person-Centered and Experiential Psychotherapies, 12*, 14–30.

Elliott, R., & Greenberg, L. S. (2007). *The essence of process-experiential: Emotion-focused therapy. American Journal of Psychotherapy, 61*(3), 241–254.

Evans, K. M., Kincade, E. A., & Seem, S. R. (2011). *Introduction to feminist therapy: Strategies for social and individual change.* Thousand Oaks, CA: Sage.

Foucault, M. (1979). *Discipline and punish* (A. Sheridan, Trans.). New York, NY: Vintage.

Fox, D., Prilleltensky, I., & Austin, S. (2009). Critical psychology for social justice: Concerns and dilemmas. In D. Fox, I. Prilleltensky, & S. Austin (Eds.), *Critical psychology: An introduction* (2nd. ed., pp. 3–19). London: Sage.

Freedman, J., & Combs, G. (1996). *Narrative therapy: The social construction of preferred realities*. New York, NY: Norton.
Garfinkel, H. (1967). *Studies in ethnomethodology*. Englewood Cliffs, NJ: Prentice-Hall.
Gilbert, P., & Leahy, R. L. (2007). Introduction and overview: Basic issues in the therapeutic relationship. In P. Gilbert & R. L. Leahy (Eds.), *The therapeutic relationship in the cognitive behavioral psychotherapies* (pp. 3–23). London: Routledge.
Goldman, R., & Greenberg, L. S. (2013). Working with identity and self-soothing in emotion-focused therapy for couples. *Family Process, 52*, 62–82.
Greenberg, L. S. (2014). The therapeutic relationship in emotion-focused therapy. *Psychotherapy, 51*(3), 350–357.
Greenberg, L. S. (2015). *Emotion-focused therapy: Coaching clients to work through their feelings*. Washington, DC: American Psychological Association.
Greenberg, L. S., Rice, L. N., & Elliott, R. (1993). *Facilitating emotional change: The moment-by-moment process*. New York, NY: Guilford.
Heritage, J. (1984). *Garfinkel and ethnomethodology*. New York, NY: Polity.
Heritage, J. (2013). Epistemics in conversation. In J. Sidnell & T. Stivers (Eds.), *The handbook of conversation analysis* (pp. 370–394). Malden, MA: Wiley-Blackwell.
Horvath, A. O., & Muntigl, P. (2018). The alliance as a discursive achievement: A conversation analytical perspective. In O. Smoliak & T. Strong (Eds.), *Therapy as discourse: Practice and research*. London: Palgrave Macmillan.
Knapp, S. J., VandeCreek, L. D., & Fingerhut, R. (2017). *Practical ethics for psychologists: A positive approach* (3rd. ed.). Washington, DC: American Psychological Association.
Koenig, C. J. (2011). Patient resistance as agency in treatment decisions. *Social Science and Medicine, 72*, 1105–1114.
Koocher, G. P., & Keith-Spiegel, P. (2016). Psychotherapy I: Ethical obligations of psychotherapists. In G. P. Koocher & P. Keith-Spiegel (Eds.), *Ethics in psychology and the mental health professions: Standards and cases* (pp. 59–84). New York, NY: Oxford University Press.
Kuyken, W., Padesky, C. A., & Dudley, R. (2009). *Collaborative case conceptualization: Working effectively with clients in cognitive-behavioral therapy*. New York, NY: Guilford.
Lakoff, G., & Johnson, M. (1980). *Metaphors we live by*. Chicago, IL: University of Chicago Press.
MacMartin, C. (2008). Resisting optimistic questions in narrative and solution-focused therapies. In A. Peräkylä, C. Antaki, S. Vehviläinen, & I. Leudar

(Eds.), *Conversation analysis and psychotherapy* (pp. 79–99). Cambridge, UK: Cambridge University Press.

Massfeller, H. F., & Strong, T. (2012). Clients as conversational agents. *Patient Education and Counseling, 88*(2), 196–202.

Maturana, H., & Varela, F. (1988). *The tree of knowledge.* Boston, MA: Shambhala.

McNamee, S., & Gergen, K. J. (1992). *Therapy as social construction.* London: Sage.

Muntigl, P., Knight, N., Horvath, A. O., & Watkins, A. (2012). Client attitudinal stance and therapist-client affiliation: A view from grammar and social interaction. *Research in Psychotherapy Psychopathology, Process and Outcome, 15*, 117–130.

Norcross, J. C., & Wampold, B. E. (2011). Evidence-based therapy relationships: Research conclusions and clinical practice. In J. C. Norcross (Ed.), *Psychotherapy relationships that work: Evidence-based responsiveness* (pp. 423–430). Washington, DC: American Psychological Association.

Oh, S. Y. (2006). English zero anaphora as an interactional resource. *Research on Language and Social Interaction, 38*(3), 267–302.

Pomerantz, A. (1984). Agreeing and disagreeing with assessments: Some features of preferred/dispreferred turn shapes. In J. M. Atkinson & J. Heritage (Eds.), *Structures of social action: Studies in conversation analysis* (pp. 57–101). Cambridge: Cambridge University Press.

Pomerantz, A. M., & Heritage, J. (2013). Preference. In J. Sidnell & T. Stivers (Eds.), *Handbook of conversation analysis* (pp. 210–228). New York, NY: Wiley-Blackwell.

Potter, J. (1996). *Representing reality.* London: Sage.

Potter, J., & Wetherell, M. (1987). *Discourse and social psychology: Beyond attitudes and behaviour.* London: Sage.

Raymond, G. (2003). Grammar and social organization: Yes/No interrogatives and the structure of responding. *American Sociological Review, 68*, 939–967.

Robertson, M., Morris, K., & Walter, G. (2007). Overview of psychiatric ethics V: Utilitarianism and the ethics of duty. *Australasian Psychiatry, 15*(5), 402–410.

Roy-Chowdhury, S. (2006). How is the therapeutic relationship talked into being? *Journal of Family Therapy, 28*, 153–174.

Rush, A. J. (2001). Practice guidelines and algorithms. In M. M. Weissman (Ed.), *Treatment of depression: Bridging the 21st century* (pp. 213–242). Washington, DC: American Psychiatric Association.

Sacks, H., Schegloff, E. A., & Jefferson, G. (1974). A simplest systematics for the organization of turn-taking in conversation. *Language, 50*, 696–735.

Safran, J. D., & Messer, S. B. (1997). Psychotherapy integration: A postmodern critique. *Clinical Psychology: Science and Practice, 1*(2), 140–152.

Shotter, J. (1993). *Conversational realities*. London: Sage.

Sidnell, J., & Stivers, T. (Eds.). (2013). *The handbook of conversation analysis*. Malden, MA: Wiley-Blackwell.

Stevanovic, M., & Peräkylä, A. (2012). Deontic authority in interaction: The right to announce, propose, and decide. *Research on Language and Social Interaction, 45*(3), 297–321.

Stiles, W. B. (2009). Responsiveness as an obstacle for psychotherapy outcome research: It's worse than you think. *Clinical Psychology: Science and Practice, 16*(1), 86–91.

Stivers, T. (2005). Parent resistance to physicians' treatment recommendations: One resource for initiating a negotiation of the treatment decision. *Health Communication, 18*(1), 41–74.

Stivers, T., Heritage, J., Barnes, R. K., McCabe, R., Thompson, L., & Toerien, M. (2017). Treatment recommendations as actions. *Health Communication*. https://doi.org/10.1080/10410236.2017.1350913

Strawbridge, S. (2003). Ethics, psychology and therapeutic practice. In D. Hill & C. Jones (Eds.), *Forms of ethical thinking in therapeutic practice* (pp. 1–17). Milton Keynes, UK: Open University Press.

Strong, T. (2000). Collaborative influence. *Australian and New Zealand Journal of Family Therapy, 21*(3), 144–148.

Strong, T., & Busch, R. (2013). DSM-V and evidence-based family therapy? *Australian and New Zealand Journal of Family Therapy, 34*(2), 90–103.

Strong, T., Busch, R., & Couture, S. (2008). Conversational evidence in therapeutic dialogue. *Journal of Marital and Family Therapy, 34*, 388–405.

Strong, T., Lysack, M., Smoliak, O., & Chondros, K. (2019). Considering the dialogic potentials of cognitive behavioural therapy. In D. Loewenthal & G. Proctor (Eds.), *Against and for CBT?* (2nd revised ed.). Ross-on-Wye, UK: PCCS Press.

Strong, T., & Sutherland, O. (2007). Conversational ethics in psychological dialogues: Discursive and collaborative considerations. *Canadian Psychology/Psychologie canadienne, 48*(2), 94–105.

Sutherland, O., Sametband, I., Gaete Silva, J., Couture, S. J., & Strong, T. (2013). Conversational perspective of therapeutic outcomes: The importance of preference in the development of discourse. *Counselling and Psychotherapy Research, 13*, 220–226.

Sutherland, O., & Strong, T. (2011). Therapeutic collaboration: A conversation analysis of constructionist therapy. *Journal of Family Therapy, 33*, 256–278.

Swim, S., St. George, S. A., & Wulff, D. P. (2001). Process ethics: A collaborative partnership. *Journal of Systemic Therapies, 20*, 14–24.

Tileagă, C., & Stokoe, E. (Eds.). (2016). *Discursive psychology: Classic and contemporary issues*. New York, NY: Routledge.

Tomm, K. (2003, January/February). Promoting social justice as an ethical imperative. *Family Therapy Magazine*, pp. 30–31.

Tomm, K. M. (1987). Interventive interviewing: Part I. Strategizing as a fourth guideline for the therapist. *Family Process, 26*, 2–13.

Tseliou, E. (2018). Conversation analysis, discourse analysis and psychotherapy research: Overview and methodological potential. In O. Smoliak & T. Strong (Eds.), *Therapy as discourse: Practice and research*. London: Palgrave Macmillan.

Turnbull, W. (2003). *Language in action. Psychological models of conversation*. New York, NY: Psychology Press.

Vehviläinen, S. (2008). Identifying and managing resistance in psychoanalytic interaction. In A. Peräkylä, C. Antaki, S. Vehviläinen, & I. Leudar (Eds.), *Conversation analysis and psychotherapy* (pp. 120–138). Cambridge: Cambridge University Press.

Wampold, B. E. (2015). How important are the common factors in psychotherapy? An update. *World Psychiatry, 14*(3), 270–277.

Weiste, E. (2015). Describing therapeutic projects across sequences: Balancing between supportive and disagreeing interventions. *Journal of Pragmatics, 80*, 22–43.

Weiste, E. H., Voutilainen, L. H., & Peräkylä, A. M. (2016). Epistemic asymmetries in psychotherapy interaction: Therapists' practices for displaying access to clients' inner experiences. *Sociology of Health & Illness, 38*(4), 645–661.

White, M. (2007). *Maps of narrative practice*. New York, NY: W. W. Norton.

White, M., & Epston, D. (1990). *Narrative means to therapeutic ends*. New York, NY: Norton.

Wiggins, S. (2017). *Discursive psychology: Theory, method, and applications*. London: Sage.

10

Discursive Research from an Assimilation Model Perspective

William B. Stiles

The foregoing chapters addressed the interrelated methodological, theoretical, and ethical aspects involved in a discursive approach to psychotherapy and to human relationships more broadly. They explored the phenomena of discourses, subject positioning, and interpersonal power, always attending to the fine-grained details of how language is used. My task is to comment. Elsewhere, I have argued that discursive approaches may offer a solution to serious problems with the most common (linear statistical) approaches to psychotherapy research but that more explicit attention to theory building would be desirable (Stiles, 2008). Discursive approaches have produced careful observations and powerful concepts, and these deserve a more general synthesis. A good theory is a compact, accurate summary of all the observations that have gone into it (Stiles, 2009).

W. B. Stiles (✉)
Glendale Springs, NC, USA
e-mail: stileswb@miamioh.edu

O. Smoliak, T. Strong (eds.), *Therapy as Discourse*, The Language of Mental Health,
https://doi.org/10.1007/978-3-319-93067-1_10

Assimilation and Historicity

In Chap. 1, Strong and Smoliak (2019) posed as central puzzles for this book, "what it is about talking that is curative or therapeutic. What does talking have to do with how one understands and experiences reality?" (p. xx). The assimilation model, a theory of psychological change that I have worked on (e.g., Stiles, 2011), addresses both of these puzzles, and I use it here in an attempt to pull together some of the observations and strands of thought in this book. This is not meant to test the model but rather to sketch a way of working within it. I apologize in advance for so many self-citations. My larger point is simply that discursive results are ripe for synthesis.

Experiences, Signs, and Voices

The term *assimilation* refers to assimilating previously disconnected, problematic, distressing experiences (e.g., traumatic experiences, unacceptable ways of being), integrating them and making them accessible and potentially useful to the rest of the person. Three key concepts in the assimilation model are experiences, signs, and voices. According to the model, the term experience refers to anything that is in awareness, including intentions and intentional actions as well as perceptions, thoughts, and feelings. The theory suggests that experiences leave traces in the person's nervous system. When these traces are reactivated, the person's experience is similar in some aspects to the original events.

Signs, such as words, have a concrete, observable presence in the world (e.g., vibrations in the air, marks on a page), but they also refer to private experiences of the author and addressee, the sign's meanings. In effect, signs make people's private experience observable, albeit selectively. Signs carry experience from author to addressee in this sense: if you understand what I am saying in this chapter, you are sharing my experience. Not perfectly, of course, but in part and in flavor. That is, my experience is being carried to you by the words on this page.

Internal voices are built by assimilation of traces of related experiences. The voices represent people, events, problems, and ways of being in the world that the person has encountered or experienced. When they are addressed by circumstances, the traces emerge to act and speak—hence the voice metaphor. A person can be construed as a mosaic of internal voices. Theoretically, therapeutic assimilation is accomplished by building semiotic meaning bridges between heretofore disconnected internal voices. Meaning bridges are signs that have similar meaning to author and addressee (Stiles, 2011).

Historicity

A word (or any sign) has a slightly different meaning each time it is used reflecting our changing experience. But words accumulate these meanings. Each use adds another layer. That is, a word's meaning is built from the experience of people who have used the word previously (Stiles, 2019). Here's how it works:

You learned the meaning of words from the people who used them to share their experience with you: your parents, teachers, friends, authors you read, television programs you watched, and so forth. When you understood what those people said, you had some version of their experience. So now, when you use those words to convey your experiences to others, your word's meaning is partly their experience. When your addressees understand you, they share a little bit of the experience of your parents, teachers, authors, and so forth, along with your experience. For example, the next time you use the word *sign* or *historicity*, there will be a bit of my experience tucked in.

Of course, you parents, teachers, and authors weren't the first people to use those words. Their use incorporated the experience of their parents, teachers, friends, authors, and so forth. In this way, words come to convey not only the experience of the speaker, but also something of the experience of the many previous speakers and writers who have used those words. For example, if you understand my words right now, you are sharing not only my experience but also the experience of Mikael Leiman (1992, 2011), a friend and colleague who taught me much of what I know about signs, and the experience of Mikhail Bakhtin (1986) and Lev Vygotsky (1924/1978), authors who shared their ideas about signs with him.

As a result of this historicity of signs, language incorporates great reservoirs of personal and cultural experience. Also, as a consequence of historicity (signs accumulating meaning), much of our experience is a recycling of other people's experience, passed to us by signs. Therapists draw on this when they intervene with clients. The many layers of meaning need not be consciously recognized by the speakers at the time. On the contrary, clients and therapists often say far more than they know.

To say it another way, the historicity of signs allows many voices to participate in the therapeutic dialogue. When people listen to their own words or the words of their interlocutor, they hear the voices of people who have used those words previously. The experiences of forebears who used those words and expressions can help clients and therapists articulate and understand and solve the problems they face.

The Historicity of Discourses and Subject Positions

The concept historicity points toward an account of the source and persistence of discourses: discourses are embedded in the signs, that is, in the meanings of the constituent words, stories, and actions. When people use the signs as author or addressee, they experience and enact bits of what their forebears experienced. In effect, I suggest, discourses can be understood as collections of internal voices carried by each participant. Theoretically, the physical and social context addresses relevant voices and the voices emerge to speak and act.

Subject positioning, as discussed by Avdi and Georgaca (2019) in Chap. 3, following Guilfoyle (2016), seems to describe the assignment of places within a discourse. Subject positions within discourses are distinct ways of being in relation to each other. Slipping into a position within a discourse involves using terms and expressions—and no doubt other, non-linguistic signs—that reproduce in part the actions and experiences of those who have used those signs previously. As people enact their positions, they reproduce their forebears' experience in themselves and they address and evoke voices within each other to reproduce the discourse. A person enacting (and experiencing) a particular position addresses reciprocal or complementary positions in others. So people draw each other in. Consider some of the conceptions of discourses offered by the authors:

In Chap. 2, Wahlström (2019) characterized a discourse as "an institutionalized variety of language-use, which can be identified based on choices of vocabulary, key-metaphors, grammatical constructions, etc." (p. xx). He distinguished three discourses that he observed in transcripts of individual therapies: colloquial (ordinary language, common words and expressions), medical (professional psychiatric or other medical terms), and therapeutic (words and phrases referring to specific psychological realms of cognition, emotions, and experiencing). Theoretically, the language (vocabulary, metaphors, grammatical constructions) of each of these discourses has acquired its meaning from the experience of previous users, including clients and therapists, patients and doctors, aggregated over generations of use. Using their language addresses their voices in addressee and author, who respond with more of their language.

In Chap. 5, Miller (2019) said, "A discourse is a body of resources that people use in making sense of their experiences and managing their lives. In shifting from one discourse to another, people engage different language and interpretive resources that may transform their senses of themselves and their lives" (p. xx). Historicity is a way of explaining the source of the "body of resources." It is the experiences of previous occupants of those subject positions, who used those terms and expressions to solve problems they had under similar circumstances. Simply casting problematic experiences in their terms gives access to the resources (Stiles, 2019).

In contrast to Wahlström's and Miller's relatively broad conceptions of what constitutes a discourse, Knudson-Martin et al. (2019) used the term *gender discourse* in Chap. 7 to refer to much more tightly limited segments of interaction, such as enactments of "men should be the authority" or "women should protect men from shame." Perhaps discourses can be understood as subdivisible, like interactions, allowing narrower distinctions as required. That is, each distinguishable part or subtype of a discourse may also be called a discourse. Translated into the context of the historicity account, Knudson-Martin et al.'s suggestion can be understood as suggesting that the accumulated meanings of signs can call people into enactments of quite specific activities.

Thus, the language available to perform normal social or professional tasks such as those required of being a client or a therapist, a husband or a wife, brings with it specific discourses and subject positions within the discourse. As we understand what is being said by our interlocutors and by ourselves, we experience ourselves in terms of the received meanings; we have parts of our forebears' experience. Conversely, using the language of a different position brings different experiences. As Avdi and Georgaca (2019) put it in Chap. 3, "We tell a different story of our troubles, for example, when we assume the position of a concerned parent, a troubled adolescent or a mentally ill patient" (p. xx).

More clinically, as pointed out by Knudson-Martin and her colleagues (2019), some of the problems clients bring to therapy can be understood as a mismatch between a client's own lived experience and the received subject positioning in the discourses into which he or she is thrown. As they put it, "the difficulties that clients experience are often seen to arise from the use of a limited range of culturally dominant, but pathologizing, discourses, which restrict the range of subject positions that can be adopted" (p. xx). In their example, Demetra could not comfortably adapt to the received subject position of being a mother, with what was for her a too-limited range of activities and experiences that came with it.

Power, Negotiation, and Therapeutic Impact

Insofar as discourses arise through the historicity of signs, which tend to reproduce aspects of forbears' experience, they may tend to preserve features of social organization that seem undesirable in a modern context. Among such problematic features are inflexible subject positions and inequitable distributions of power and respect. Foucauldian studies in particular have focused on ways in which power inequities in available discourses have been dysfunctional for clients. As Miller (2019, Chap. 5) and Knudson-Martin et al. (2019, Chap. 7) discussed in detail, part of the task of a discursive therapist is making changes in the discourses themselves, at least as practiced by their clients.

Theoretically, people in inequitable power relationships assimilate both roles and when called upon can enact either. Given circumstances that assign them a reciprocal subject position, people can and often do switch positions. For example, the abused can too easily become the abuser. Changing the discourse itself is more difficult, as it must overcome the inertia of historicity.

Discursive therapies typically seek to minimize power differences, both among clients (e.g., within families or couples) and between therapists and clients, resulting in an emphasis on negotiation, support for those in less powerful subject positions, and work toward more collaborative relationships both inside and outside of therapy (Knudson-Martin et al., 2019, Chap. 7; Miller, 2019, Chap. 5; Smoliak, Strong, & Elliott, 2019, Chap. 9). In Chap. 9, Smoliak et al. (2019) explicitly cast the process goal of negotiation and collaboration as a core ethical issue. They contrast these "discursive ethics" with top-down ethics they see as implicit (sometimes explicit) in the evidence-based practice (EBP) movement: that the therapist is understood as an expert whose job is to specify the means and process goals of treatment (we might say, invoking an expert-client discourse).

Discursive methods can illuminate how this is done. For example, both the enactment of power relationships and a means of negotiation are illustrated by reflexive questions, as described by Gaete Silva, Smoliak, and Couture (2019) in Chap. 6. These are formally (grammatically) questions but have an additional function, such as indirectly advancing ("referring, hinting, evoking," p. xx) a therapeutic interpretation or therapeutic advice. "[T]hey help craft and invite continued co-constructed distinctions and meanings regarded as more preferable or helpful as compared to prior meanings" (p. xx). In some cases, the additional function may be the therapist's intent (on record or off record; Stiles, 1986). In other cases, the therapist's intention may be a pure question, but the frame of reference in which the question is framed (i.e., the therapist's) nevertheless has the effect of redirecting the client's understanding or action. Thus, reflexive questions represent an exercise of the therapist's power. On the other hand, because the question form is less presumptuous than a bald interpretation or directive would be (Stiles, 1992), it allows more leeway for negotiation. The content is perhaps more likely to be worked with, and perhaps to help facilitate self-healing.

The Power of Discursive Methods

The particular strength of discursive methods has been to demonstrate the importance of fine details in human interaction, as illustrated by the observations of systematically unequal power in relationships. Discursive approaches, with their emphasis on the actions performed by language, what is done rather than what is said (cf. Austin, 1975), are well suited to unpacking how such relational features as power and intimacy enacted in, for example, therapist-client relationships and relationships within couples (Avdi & Georgaca, 2019, Chap. 3; Knudson-Martin et al., 2019, Chap. 7) and families (Horvath & Muntigl, 2019, Chap. 4).

As Horvath and Muntigl (2019) noted in Chap. 4, human interaction is characterized by ubiquitous responsiveness. People in psychotherapy, and indeed in any conversation, are always responding to each other on time scales ranging from months to milliseconds. From the perspective of traditional statistical hypothesis-testing research in psychotherapy research, this responsiveness entails reciprocal dependence of psychotherapy process variables on any timescale greater than milliseconds and thus violates basic independence assumptions. By contrast, discursive approaches to research, such as conversation analysis (CA), make responsive processes their main topic of study.

> The detailed "microscopic" attention to conversational elements also enable us to track how "appropriate responsiveness," doing the right thing at the right time (Stiles & Horvath, 2017), is realized in a clinical situation. (Horvath & Muntigl, 2019, p. xx)

Horvath and Muntigl used CA techniques to unpack responsiveness in the crucial therapeutic task of building a strong alliance. Such techniques are likewise well suited to unpacking the building of semiotic meaning bridges and the manifestations of historicity. In

Chap. 5, Miller (2019) reviewed CA, ethnomethodology, and Foucauldian studies as approaches that can deal with responsiveness by looking closely at the details of dialogue and interpersonal interaction. As Tseliou (2019) put it in Chap. 8:

> CA and DPsy [discursive psychology] bear the methodological potential for the study of the process of change by locating analysis within *in situ*, *interdependent* sequences which are simultaneously studied from participants' perspective without resorting to post-session reports or narrations about therapy. (p. xx)

Concluding Comments

This commentary's account of discourses as a product of historicity is a new extension of the assimilation model, not something previously addressed. It is generally consistent with previous assimilation theory and observation, but it involves new theoretical proposals. This sort of incremental modification of the theory is central to theory building, an expectable consequence of a theory encountering new observations (Rennie, 2012; Stiles, 2009).

Historicity is not destiny. According to the theory, we add to a word's meaning each time we say it. Sign meanings derive from previous uses, but they change every time they are used. Anyone who communicates is adding their own experience to the pool of meaning carried by the language they use. If a discursive therapy client achieves a more satisfying life or a more caring relationship or a more equal subject position, the improved discourse becomes embedded in the signs it uses, and those signs can help others who come later.

References

Avdi, E., & Georgaca, E. (2019). Researching the discursive construction of subjectivity in psychotherapy. In T. Strong & J. O. Smoliak (Eds.), *Therapy as discourse*. Basingstoke, UK: Palgrave Macmillan.

Austin, J. L. (1975). *How to do things with words* (2nd ed.). Oxford: Clarendon Press.

Bakhtin, M. M. (1986). *Speech genres and other late essays*. Austin, TX: University of Texas Press.

Gaete Silva, J., Sutherland, O., & Couture, S. (2019). Reflexive questions as constructive interventions: A discursive perspective. In T. Strong & J. O. Smoliak (Eds.), *Therapy as discourse*. Basingstoke, UK: Palgrave Macmillan.

Guilfoyle, M. (2016). Subject positioning: Gaps and stability in the therapeutic encounter. *Journal of Constructivist Psychology, 29*(2), 123–140.

Horvath, A. O., & Muntigl, P. (2019). The alliance as a discursive achievement: A conversation analytical perspective. In T. Strong & J. O. Smoliak (Eds.), *Therapy as discourse*. Basingstoke, UK: Palgrave Macmillan.

Knudson-Martin, C., ChenFeng, J., Galick, A., Lobo, E., Samman, S. K., & Williams, K. (2019). Transforming gender discourse in couple therapy: Researching intersections of societal discourse, emotion, and interaction. In T. Strong & J. O. Smoliak (Eds.), *Therapy as discourse*. Basingstoke, UK: Palgrave Macmillan.

Leiman, M. (1992). The concept of sign in the work of Vygotsky, Winnicott, and Bakhtin: Further integration of object relations theory and activity theory. *British Journal of Medical Psychology, 65*, 209–222.

Leiman, M. (2011). Michael Bakhtin's contribution to psychotherapy research. *Culture & Psychology, 17*, 441–461.

Miller, G. (2019). Discursive therapies as institutional discourse. In T. Strong & J. O. Smoliak (Eds.), *Therapy as discourse*. Basingstoke, UK: Palgrave Macmillan.

Rennie, D. L. (2012). Qualitative research as methodical hermeneutics. *Psychological Methods, 17*, 385–398. https://doi.org/10.1037/a0029250

Smoliak, O., Strong, T., & Elliott, R. (2019). Discursive ethics in therapeutic encounters. In T. Strong & J. O. Smoliak (Eds.), *Therapy as discourse*. Basingstoke, UK: Palgrave Macmillan.

Stiles, W. B. (1986). Levels of intended meaning of utterances. *British Journal of Clinical Psychology, 25*, 213–222.

Stiles, W. B. (1992). *Describing talk: A taxonomy of verbal response modes*. Newbury Park, CA: Sage.

Stiles, W. B. (2008). Foreword: Filling the gaps. In A. Peräkylä, C. Antaki, S. Vehviläinen, & I. Leudar (Eds.), *Conversation analysis and psychotherapy* (pp. 1–4). Cambridge, UK: Cambridge University Press.

Stiles, W. B. (2009). Logical operations in theory-building case studies. *Pragmatic Case Studies in Psychotherapy, 5*(3), 9–22. https://doi.org/10.14713/pcsp.v5i3.973 Retrieved from http://jrul.libraries.rutgers.edu/index.php/pcsp/article/view/973

Stiles, W. B. (2011). Coming to terms. *Psychotherapy Research, 21*, 367–384. https://doi.org/10.1080/10503307.2011.582186

Stiles, W. B. (2019). Assimilation of problematic voices and the historicity of signs: How culture enters psychotherapy. In A. Konopka, H. Hermans, & M. Goncalves (Eds.), *Dialogical self theory: Bridging psychotherapeutic traditions and cultural contexts.* London: Routledge.

Stiles, W. B., & Horvath, A. O. (2017). Appropriate responsiveness as a contribution to therapist effects. In L. Castonguay & C. E. Hill (Eds.), *How and why are some therapists better than others? Understanding therapist effects* (pp. 71–84). Washington, DC: APA Books.

Strong, T., & Smoliak, O. (2019). Introduction to discursive research and discursive therapies. In T. Strong & J. O. Smoliak (Eds.), *Therapy as discourse.* Basingstoke, UK: Palgrave Macmillan.

Tseliou, E. (2019). Conversation analysis, discourse analysis and psychotherapy research: Overview and methodological potential. In T. Strong & J. O. Smoliak (Eds.), *Therapy as discourse.* Basingstoke, UK: Palgrave Macmillan.

Vygotsky, L. S. (1924/1978). *Mind and society: The development of higher psychological processes.* Cambridge, MA: Harvard University Press (Original work published 1924).

Wahlström, J. (2019). Discourse in psychotherapy—Using words to create therapeutic practice. In T. Strong & J. O. Smoliak (Eds.), *Therapy as discourse.* Basingstoke, UK: Palgrave Macmillan.

Appendix

Table A.1 Conversation analytic transcription conventions

(.5)	Silence represented in tenths of a second
(.)	Hearable silence that is less than two-tenths of a second
=	Latching
-	Cut-off
( )	Material in parentheses is inaudible
(( ))	Comments of the researcher
:	The prolongation or stretching of the sound just preceding it (one or more colons)
Under	Words that were uttered with added emphasis
CAPITAL	Words were uttered louder than the surrounding talk
hhh	Hearable aspiration (laughter, breathing)
.hhh	Inhalation of breath
heh	Laughter
?	Strongly rising intonation
.	A falling intonation contour
,	Slightly rising intonation
¿	Pitch rise that is stronger than a comma but weaker than a question mark
° °	Talk between ° ° is quieter than surrounding talk
><	Talk between >< is quicker than surrounding talk
[ ]	Overlap of talk
↓	Downward shift in pitch

O. Smoliak, T. Strong (eds.), *Therapy as Discourse*, The Language of Mental Health,
https://doi.org/10.1007/978-3-319-93067-1

↓	Upward shift in pitch
~	Tremulous voice
--->	The action described continues across subsequent lines

Note: Adapted from "Transcribing for social research" by A. Hepburn and G. Bolden, 2017

Index[1]

[1] Note: Page numbers followed by 'n' refer to notes.

O. Smoliak, T. Strong (eds.), *Therapy as Discourse*, The Language of Mental Health,
https://doi.org/10.1007/978-3-319-93067-1